I0439205

ABC
water

and the

Number Crunch Diet

Jumper Publications and Media

DEDICATION

This book is dedicated to all the authors whose books have helped me to understand science, diet, lifestyle, fitness, wellness and selfcare. Many of these people are not household names, some of them have even passed on, but their insight, discoveries, and commitment to helping others through their writings lives on, sadly however, some of it lives on attached to other people's names, but, none-the-less, these unsung heroes, the original authors, will no doubt hear, "Well done thou good and faithful servant."

Disclaimer

The purpose of this book is to empower the reader with knowledge, to educate, informational purposes. This book is not medical advice, but rather the author's personal experience, and is a guide for anyone who wishes to implement said dietary or lifestyle changes at the reader's own discretion. The choice between medical care and self care is completely up to the reader. If you have a medical problem, seek medical care. The author and Jumper Publications and Media shall not be held responsible or liable for any and all damages, loss, or injury, of any kind that may be caused or allegedly caused, directly or indirectly, by the information in this book. Reading beyond this page is the reader's consent to the above disclaimer.

CONTENTS

Acknowledgment

Thought

In a world where freethinking has never been so great, there are elements of society, powers, that would like to shape it to their advantage, truth or no truth. There's a saying that goes, "You'll know it when you see it." Some things, you just know. I never let anyone THINK for me. I never let ANYONE think for me. I NEVER LET anyone think for me.

When I was a kid, I can recall a jingle from a TV commercial for a board game, and it went, "The game of life." The board game was called "Life". Other games I recall playing were "Monopoly" "Clue" "Operation". Putting them all together, one could ask, "Do you have a Clue about the game of Life run by a Monopoly that if you are not careful could result in your needing an Operation?"

There's a story of two men, one had money and the other had wisdom. When the two men got together, interacted, and departed, the man with the money had the wisdom, and the man with the wisdom had the money.

I would like to thank the wise people, who, through their good advice, steered me in the right direction, keeping me from harm's way. I would also like to thank my Creator, God, and for his Angels, upon which my faith has been built.

But without faith it is impossible to please him:
For he that cometh to God must believe that he is,
and that he is a rewarder of them that diligently seek him.

Hebrews 11.6

To purchase additional copies, please visit

http://www.CreateSpace.com/4739779

Edits & Format

You will notice oddities in punctuation, spelling, syntax, and perhaps even semantics, within this book. Feel free to let me know, but some of it is done for brevity or to shift emphasis. I use capitals where I see fit, to grab your attention and make it stand out, and I also remove capitals when I don't think they are deserving of them, or to remove emphasis after first usage, i.e., Pyrex becomes pyrex. And french bread, brussels sprouts, and english cucumbers, are spelled lowercase, as we are not going to "link" a European vacation to our food and eating.

Secondly, I will unhyphenate to create rhythm. Grammatically, two or more words that function as an adjective before a noun are supposed to be hyphenated. That's fine. A million-dollar smile, is the adjective "million-dollar" describing the smile. However, this can get redundant after a while, 1&2 3, 1&2 3, 1&2 3. The noun gets all the attention. But what if you want the adjectives to have the emphasis? After all, the adjectives are the descriptive words. So, I will drop the hyphens to allow the adjectives equal emphasis, and to change the pace of the sentence a bit. So if there are no hyphens, read it slower and evenly, one two three four five six seven. A "step-by-step solution" sounds a bit skippy and simplistic, whereas, a "step by step solution" is said slower and sounds more methodical. Hyphenating two words, or joining two words as a compound word, reduces their individual meanings.

With regard to fastfood, healthfood, and seasalt, it's time for these words to evolve into compound words, so the trend starts here.

There are also some fragmented sentences, subject-verb disagreements, and singular/plural violations. When "correcting" certain of these sentences, they lost their emphasis and punch, so I kept them as is.

In the past I've been guilty of judging other author's sentences, only to reread it with the commas, pauses, and then it made perfect sense. So, if there's a comma, then pause, as you may not get to pause later in the sentence. If there's no comma, then don't pause and read it all as one.

I pose questions, but without question marks. Some are rhetorical, but some are to make you Ponder. Great word. Ponder. If you see a question mark at the end, then it requires an answer. If there's no question mark, then you can just say, yeah, no, or hm.

English continues to change, people using it, customize the language to fit what they want to communicate, emphasize, and to make their point from various angles. It also has to have a variety of melodies and rhythms to keep it from being boring. If you find yourself having to reread a sentence, it may be that it's structured that way for that very reason. So take your time. Don't rush. Let the words digest, so that you absorb the material, and hopefully take some of it and make it a part of your life.

Lastly, you will notice that I customized the headers of every page! This is not something Microsoft Word Starter allows you to do. You can only customize three pages, first, even, and odd. So, to get around this I had to create a Page Break every three pages, and as a result, the last line of some of the pages doesn't "justify" to the edge. So I hope that flipping through the upper corners of the pages will assist you in finding the chapter that you are looking for.

You won't see any citations from scientific studies or PubMed, because at JPM we look to a higher source for our reference.

God Bless!

Enjoy the Journey

Email me if you have a question, or if you just want to comment. Your purchase comes with 2-years free support and photos.

Barry Ogston, B.Sc., CLS, MLS(ASCP)

You have to crunch the numbers to see what you're really eating.

CHAPTER 1

INTRODUCTION

Hi! And welcome to Jumper Publications and Media™.

A jumper is a device that connects one wire on a circuit board to another wire on a circuit board, allowing for – The Transfer of Information From One to the Other.

Jumper Publications share personal experiences and unique knowledge of dietary and lifestyle changes that resulted in improved health, energy, and fitness level. They cut through all the general advice such as "exercise" "lose weight" "eat more omega-3s and less omega-6s" "keep your body slightly alkaline" et cetera, and show you EXACTLY how to do it. Expect a lot of detail, as Jumper Publications are the only books that I am aware of that give you EVERYTHING you need to make this particular lifestyle or dietary change. All the searching and researching, reading, experimenting, trial and error have been done. Many many hours have been spent figuring out and perfecting the dietary or lifestyle change so that the reader and other likeminded people can have the bottom line "How To".

There is no pressure to take this advice. You are a free agent and able to make your own choices. Jumper Publications and Media make no claims that you will experience any of the benefits that the author has experienced from drinking ABC Water™ or from the Number Crunch Diet™ plan. Additionally, we are not recommending that you do anything stated on the following pages. To do so would be irresponsible and reckless as we have never seen you or talked to you and every person is unique in their size, weight, genetics, body chemistry, and health. Any decision to implement a JPM lifestyle or dietary change is 100% your own choice. We simply show you how it can be done, step by step, in full detail. Jumper Publications and the author are not liable for any harm or damages arising from the contents of its publications. Reading beyond this page is your consent and agreement to the above disclaimer.

We also include some of the benefits of the lifestyle or dietary change, benefit claims which are published in the literature, on television, and widely accepted as true. For example, everyone agrees that you need to keep your body slightly alkaline because the normal pH of the blood is 7.4. To be textbook specific, the normal range for your blood is 7.35 to 7.45, so 7.4 is right in the middle. We are not making this claim, it is written in textbooks. Some claims are unique to JPM and may not be agreed upon by all, such as stating that it is wise to provide your body with a steady supply of the water-soluble vitamins B and C. While we believe this to be good advice, there are those that still cling to the old adage that, "Vitamins just create expensive urine." It is up to the reader to decide what's best for him or herself and proceed accordingly.

Lastly, as of this date, JPM and its author have no affiliations or receive any financial support from any of the companies mentioned in this publication. However, should any support be offered, it would be accepted and used to provide more publications and to reach more readers. I encourage you to support us in this mission. Thank you.

Let's begin!

CHAPTER 2

OVERVIEW

When I looked at all the habits of good health that I currently do, I made a Top Ten List. Resveratrol is not in the number one spot. Although it has valid claims as a supplement, and I personally have two bottles in my refrigerator, it didn't make the top 10. Neither did Chromium Picolinate, or CoQ10, or Ashwagandha, all of which are valid at some level, but the danger of them is that they sidetrack you from that which is most important. It's like going to Walmart to buy chrome polish for your car rims when your transmission fluid is black. Clearly, there are more important things one should be doing. What did make the top ten list, and in the number one spot is, ABC WATER™.

ABC stands for Alkaline, Vitamin B, Vitamin C. Now instinctively you should see that this is a good thing.

Alkaline water is absolutely what you should be drinking. Many bottled waters that I have purchased and tested had a pH of 6, 5.5, and even 5. This is acid water. This publication will show you how to make your water alkaline.

Of the five vitamins, ABCDE, only B and C are water-soluble. You get the oil-soluble A, D, and E, from your food, supplements added to your food, and in the case of D, sunlight as well. Vitamin K is also an oil-soluble vitamin, but it's not routinely supplemented and you should be getting it from leafy greens.

So B and C are your two water-soluble vitamins and are absolutely essential. A vitamin, by definition, is a nutrient molecule that our bodies cannot make, so we have to consume them. Oil-soluble vitamins do get stored in the body, like how you would store food items in your pantry, so they're there when you need them. But B and C get washed out into the urine, there isn't a lot stored, so a steady supply of these two vitamins is best.

Minerals are critical as well. They did make the top ten list, but will be addressed in a separate publication.

Lastly, I will explain how to determine your current level of alkalinity (or acidity) by wetting a small piece of pH paper with your urine and comparing the color to the color chart. This is very exciting, because this is how I came to understand my health status better. Just briefly, whenever I felt fatigued, my urine pH was 5, acidic. Consuming 8 sips, about 8 ounces of ABC Water, made me feel better within a few minutes. Before long, I recognized that when that feeling of fatigue hit, sure enough, my urine pH was 5. Then, I got ahead of the game. I started paying closer attention to my body's fatigue signs. Instead of waiting for fatigue to hit me, I paid attention to it sneaking up on me. So, at the first signs of fatigue, a little sore feet, some slight eyelid droop, energy starting to crash, a desire to sit down instead of move, I would check my urine pH and it would be 6. So, I know what 5 feels like, and now I know what 6 feels like. Later on, when I got my body's alkaline stores stocked up and my urine pH to stay at 7, I recognized a correlation, that being, 7 feels great, 6 is okay, 5 is yucky. There is some work involved, but the benefit far exceeds the work. Fast-forward, I no longer take my urine pH because I know exactly how much ABC Water to drink each day to maintain adequate alkalinity, and how much additional ABC Water I need if I perform physical work, such as yardwork, running, or working out. The fatigue from physical activity is in part due to the acid, and the sooner you mop it up the better you will feel.

This Acid Alkaline concept, and keeping your body slightly alkaline and preventing it from becoming acidic, is in the

NUMBER ONE spot of my top ten list.

"And the number one thing you or I or anyone else should be doing is…drumroll…Keeping Your Body pH Slightly Alkaline and Avoid Becoming Acidic."

Look forward to learning how your body feels when your urine pH is 5, 6, and 7. Make the ABC Water according to the recipe and notice the change in how you feel when you bump your urine pH up from 5 to 6 to 7.

Chapter Endnote
The dictionary lists "drinking water" as a two word noun, water fit for drinking. However, I have hyphenated it to avoid reading it as "drinking" the verb and "water" the noun. If you read it as a unit "drinking-water" the sentences flow nicely. The same applies to "reverse osmosis". It simply flows better with a hyphen, when used before a noun. I was surprise to see "water-soluble" and "oil-soluble" as permanently hyphenated words in the dictionary, hyphenated when used as a compound adjective but also hyphenated when used as a noun.

CHAPTER 3

THE A

To alkalize your drinking-water we will be using bicarbonate, specifically, a combination of sodium bicarbonate and potassium bicarbonate.

For the sodium bicarbonate, go to your local healthfood store or good-quality supermarket and buy Baking Soda in the baking aisle. Don't buy baking soda in the cleaning-products section, this is industrial grade and not food grade.

The baking soda I buy is from Trader Joe's Supermarket, it's Trader Joe's brand, 12oz 340g costs $0.99, and it has one ingredient, sodium bicarbonate USP. So this baking soda is a grade above food grade, it's United States Pharmacopeia standards, the highest available grade.

Don't buy any baking soda that lists aluminum. This is a metal used to make planes, not a nutrient required by the body.

You will add 2.5 level measuring teaspoons to one gallon of water to make the ABC Water.

A measuring teaspoon is of course NOT the same as a teaspoon used to eat dessert or stir your coffee. And "level" means you swipe the back of a knife across the measuring spoon to flatten or level it. Also, notice I didn't say a "packed down" level measuring teaspoon. Just, scoop and swipe, twice with the 1t and once with the ½t = 2½t.

For the potassium bicarbonate I chose www.nuts.com (800) 558-6887. Type "potassium bicarbonate" in the search-box and there it is. It's $6.99 per pound. If you buy five or more it's $6.78/lb. I purchased 6 lbs, which came as six one-pound bags, so I only have one bag open while the other bags stay sealed. The ingredient on the bag says "potassium bicarbonate". It doesn't say what grade, but the web page says it's food grade. The shipping was $10.35 UPS ground, and the total came to $51.03. You will use 2½ level measuring teaspoons per gallon of ABC Water.

In total, we have five level measuring teaspoons per gallon, 2½t sodium bicarbonate and 2½t potassium bicarbonate.

Now, you will want to check the pH of the drinking-water you will be using. The drinking-water I use is reverse-osmosis tap water and its pH is 5. It takes 1t bicarbonate to raise the pH of my drinking-water from 5 to 7.5. This would be appropriate for me if I had been a vegetarian for the past ten years and had been eating an alkaline diet of 100% plant foods, but I wasn't, and I don't currently. My current diet consists of about 30% protein, acid producing, and I do hard physical work three times a week, acid producing, and I eat about three servings of fruits and vegetables, alkaline producing, on average per day. So my alkaline consumption of dietary plants, is not sufficient for my acid production from dietary protein and physical exercise. I need to supplement.

So, five teaspoons bicarbonate per gallon, one teaspoon just to get my drinking-water up from 5 to 7.5, that leaves four teaspoons bicarbonate supplementation per gallon, or one teaspoon bicarbonate per quart.

If your drinking-water is pH 7, terrific, perhaps you live out in the country, or, I do know that a certain water-bottling company's five-gallon Spring Water is pretty close to pH 7. If this is the case, then use 2t sodium bicarbonate and 2t potassium bicarbonate per gallon.

If your drinking-water is pH 6, use 2.25t sodium bicarbonate and 2.25t potassium bicarbonate.

Now, you may not need to supplement with bicarbonate. As stated, if you've been a vegan for the past ten years your alkaline status is likely to be fine, but I can't say anything about you personally because I do not know you personally. I can only tell you what I do, and what I can reasonably generalize about others.

Here's an added twist though, and it's called mental stress. The kind that rolls around in your head day and night. Examples would be, you're going through a messy divorce, you have a boss who's corrupt and wants you gone, you have stress from your teenagers, you have financial worries, legal worries, business worries. Anything that is on your mind 24/7. This type of stress is the worst of all acid-producers. With dietary protein, you eat it, it gets metabolized, burned, and leaves behind acid, and it's done. With exercise, you do it, and in the process of pushing your muscles they create acid, and then you stop exercising and the acid production slows to a stop. However, replaying mental stress over and over in your head produces a never-ending 24/7 supply of acid. This is the worst source of acid, because it doesn't stop. This is why people can look unwell during a messy divorce, or when their business is going under, or when they just don't know how they are going to get out of a messy messy life situation. They are in a state of acidosis. Top that with the usual abandonment of a healthy diet during times of stress, it is no surprise that during the trial or shortly thereafter the person develops signs of aging.

I say, mental stress is deadly. And we've all been through it at some point in our lives. Cope the best you can, stay professional and refrain from fighting back in a wrong way, and maintain good healthy habits of diet, exercise, sleep, hydration, and ABC Water. Lock in to your Faith, your Creator, a higher power than yourself, but be alert to twists and turns and act accordingly to hold your ground. If in the end you lose, learn something from it.

Remember, King Solomon asked God for understanding and the ability to discern, and it pleased God, and God gave it to him. He will do it for you as well in your time of trial. With wisdom you have everything you need to do all else. Vitamin B is great for stress, and B and C together is even better. Be aware that the life trial is creating acid via mental turmoil and, if it was me, I would supplement with additional alkalinity to keep it mopped up on a real-time basis. You don't want to tap into your alkaline stores if you don't need to. You want to save that for a disaster, recovering from a car accident, or some other emergency situation.

In conclusion then, if you've been a vegetarian for the past ten years, but, you find yourself in a life situation with 24/7 mental stress that's been going on for weeks or months, you probably need to supplement with bicarbonate.

The only way to know is to check your urine pH, every urination for a week, and I'll talk more on this later and provide some examples.

The take-home message of this chapter is, the A part of the ABC Water recipe is 2.5t sodium bicarb and 2.5t potassium bicarb per gallon, if your drinking-water is pH 5. For drinking-water that's pH 6, drop it to 2.25t and 2.25t. And if your drinking-water is pH 7, use 2t and 2t.

If this whole pH thing has you confused, hang in there, I'll explain it more as we go along. If this is too basic for you and you're bored, sit tight, it gets better.

Chapter Endnote
Coming up, you are going to see "less-than" and "greater-than". Initially, I spelled them as two separate words, but when I saw Wikipedia spelling them with hyphens, it occurred to me that, yes, we say it as a unit, and it sounds better as "lessthan" rather than "less than". Grammarians will disagree, oh well.

CHAPTER 4

THE B

The vitamin B will be in the form of B complex, the eight primary B vitamins, thiamine (B1), riboflavin (B2), niacinamide (B3), pantothenic acid (B5), pyridoxine (B6), biotin (B7), folic acid (B9), and everyone's favorite cyanocobalamin (B12). You need all the B vitamins, and ideally, in a steady stream, rather than a once-a-day dose.

Here's where I purchase mine, and suggest you do too because vitamin B can taste bad if you don't buy a pure brand, and then your ABC Water won't taste good.

www.drclarkstore.com   ph: (866) 372-5275 or (866) DrClark. This supplement company is unique in that it prides itself on selling PURE supplements. No fillers, no colors, no binders, no coatings, no magnesium stearate, not now, not ever. Their supplements are clean. I read the label on a supplement bottle at a discount store once and the list of chemical additives was just awful. The healthfood store has good brands, but still, additives are listed on the bottles of many of their products. Dr. Clark Store is the leader in PURITY in my opinion, and this is in fact their company's slogan. I believe they were also the originators of the Purity Movement, and now you may notice other companies and brands are using the word "Purity" in their advertising because people want pure products. You can taste the difference, and how it passes through your digestive system. There is another company that I buy from that sells pure supplements with no additives, and I purchase magnesium, zinc, and vitamin E from them, and I will share this website with you later.

If you plan on drinking ABC Water every day like I do, then you'll want the purest products on the market, otherwise, you could potentially be doing more harm than good by exposing yourself to a daily dose of trace contaminants.

Order the Super B100. It currently costs $20.89 for 100 capsules. You will be able to make 100 gallons of ABC Water with one bottle of B100, using one capsule per gallon. The cost works out to $0.21 per gallon, or about five cents per quart. If you drink one quart of ABC Water per day, then you'll be spending less-than six cents per day to ensure that your bloodstream has a steady supply of all the essential B vitamins.

DrClarkStore.com offers free shipping when you order $150 or more, so I place my order once a year and pay no shipping. Additionally, once a year they send me a 20%-off coupon in the mail and this is when I place my annual order. So, free shipping and 20% off drops the price down to about one cent per eight ounces of ABC Water. Where's the expensive urine, I don't see any.

I drink one quart of ABC Water a day religiously. For every 30 minutes of hard physical work, such as running or weightlifting, or 60 minutes of moderate physical work, like yardwork or washing the car, I add another half quart. Each person has to determine for themselves how much alkaline supplementation is needed to keep your body alkaline and to prevent tapping into your alkaline stores. If you run deficient on a daily basis, then eventually you'll use up all your alkaline stores. The classic sign of this is urine that smells like Ammonia. I will explain this more later, but if your urine smells like ammonia, your body is running on the emergency back-up alkaline system. This is serious. If this is you, I would start eating more vegetables ASAP. Carrot juice, carrots and greens, carrots greens and beets, beets and apple, apple and pear, whatever is fresh and ideally organic, just get more vegetables and fruits, and cut back on the protein and hard physical work.

A healthy 20-year-old vegetarian who doesn't work out hard probably doesn't need any additional alkalinity. It is up to the reader to determine his or her current acid or alkaline status and then determine how much additional alkalinity he or she needs to get your stores stocked up and then how much you need daily for maintenance. I will expand on this more later on, so no worries, I won't leave you hangin'.

To conclude, 100 gallons is 400 quarts, therefore, I use about one bottle of Super B100 per year. What better way to ensure that I have a steady stream of all the essential B vitamins every day 365 days a year.

CHAPTER 5

THE C

Vitamin C is your body's primary water-soluble antioxidant, combatting the aging effects of free-radical damage, or, "rust". It also plays a role in collagen formation, for tighter skin, and helps heal tissues everywhere in the body. I love vitamin C.

You need vitamin C daily, and a steady supply is best.

I purchase this at DrClarkStore.com, again, for purity reasons. You have two choices. I buy the Vitamin C Powder and use 1/2 a level measuring teaspoon per gallon of ABC Water. Alternatively, you could buy the capsules, and use 2 caps per gallon.

The powder costs $19.79 for 454 grams (g), one pound (lb). The capsules cost $10.99 for 100 capsules. On the surface, the capsules look like the better deal, but let's crunch the numbers.

The capsules are 1000mg each, which is milligrams, or $1/1000^{th}$ of a gram. To convert to grams, you divide milligrams by 1000, hence 1000mg = 1g. So, 100 capsules times 1g = 100g of vitamin C for $10.99. Next, in order to compare the cost of this to the powder we need to adjust it to 454g and crunch it, 454g divided by 100g = 4.54, times $10.99 = $49.89. So, the powder at $19.79 per 454g is less-than half the price of the capsules at $49.89 per 454g.

None-the-less, some of you may not want to deal with measuring out a half teaspoon of the powder and would rather just open two capsules and add them in. I buy the powder.

Adding a ½t of vitamin-C powder to one gallon of water provides 570mg of vitamin C per quart. If you use two capsules, you will have 500mg per quart. Either way is fine.

There are 172 servings of ½t vitamin-C powder in the 1lb 454g container. That makes 172 gallons of ABC Water, so this will last me about 1.75 years. The cost then, with my 20%-off coupon and free shipping comes out to less-than 2½ cents per quart, or less-than a penny per eight ounces.

So the cost of my ABC Water for the vitamin B and vitamin C is a whopping $0.02 per eight ounce glass. And this is using the purest supplements available.

I am currently thinking of doubling, tripling, or even quadrupling the amount of vitamin C on the days that I work out, to neutralize free-radical damage from the workout and speed up recovery. On workout days, I may add an additional ½t, (double), or an additional 1t, (triple), the amount of vitamin C. I think that would be wise, as hard physical work creates a flood of free-radical damage, and the sooner I get recovered from a workout the better.

Okay! We have all of our ABC ingredients!

Sodium Bicarb	2.5t
Potassium Bicarb	2.5t
Super B100	1cap
Vitamin C Powder	½t

Now we need the water!

CHAPTER 6

THE WATER

Everyone seems to have their own opinions and ideas about what type of water is acceptable to drink. What I am about to say here is consistent with what informed people believe. If any of it offends you, don't be offended, just think about it.

Top-of-the-list don'ts is, don't drink bottled water from soft-plastic water bottles. At one time I did this, and soon came to realize that the water tasted dead, and even bad. Soft plastics leach. And one of the properties of water is that it likes to "pick up" things, chemicals. It's a dissolver. A solvent. You put something into water and the water molecules eat away at it, breaking it up and spreading it out. On a small scale this happens at the interior surface of the plastic water bottle. Now, you might think, "I'm not worried about trace amounts of BPA," bisphenol A, the chemical that made the news, and was then banned from infant baby bottles. But, try this. The next hot day in the summer, take your one-liter or 16oz bottle of soft-plastic water, and leave it on the seat of your car while you are at work. At the end of your shift, crack it open and drink it.

This is where there's a "brain washing" effect going on. I have a family member who has fantastic delicious pure tap water that comes down from the snowcapped mountains, and they were drinking 16oz bottles of soft-plastic water by the 24-pack case. When I asked, "Why are you drinking bottled water, when you know that soft plastics leach, and when you have delicious pure tap water?" The reply was, "I duh no." Duh is right. You have to think about everything you do. Are you doing it by your own choice, or are you doing it because everyone else is doing it, also referred to as "Herd Mentality", or are you doing it because you saw an advertisement, or you saw that advertisement 100+ times, "Repetitive Conditioning".

Here is my challenge to you. Go through your day and ask yourself, "Am I consciously making my own choices, or am I making choices on Autopilot, without really thinking about them?"

Plastic chemicals, like BPA, that get into the body disrupt the body's hormonal system. So the next time you hear someone say, "She has a hormonal imbalance," or your doctor tells you that he thinks your symptoms "could be due to a hormonal imbalance," THINK PLASTICS. Remove soft plastics from your life, and never never eat hot food or liquids from a soft-plastic container.

When I buy milk or orange juice, the first thing I do after I open it is transfer the entire contents to glass. In the 1950s milk used to be bottled in glass. In the 1990s, ketchup and mustard used to come in glass. Soft plastics have invaded our lives, and the health consequences have only recently been seen in their ability to enter the baby from the plastic feeding bottle.

There is a doctor who coined the term "Gender Bending Plastics" because of the hormonal effect plastic chemicals like BPA, and phthalates, have on the pregnant mother's system. All human fetuses begin as a female, and if they have two X sex chromosomes, then they stay a female. If the fetus has one X and one Y chromosome, then the female fetus is scheduled to become a male during the first trimester. The mother's hormones stimulate the baby to produce testosterone, resulting in male genitalia and a male brain. Men are providers, women are nurturers, men are protectors, women are supporters, and on and on. A man brain is, or should be, different from a woman brain, despite certain efforts from our culture to make us all the same. So your boy grows up to be sort of soft, and lacks that certain "machismo" quality. These "soft" effeminate men are going to end up having a hard time in life. Men don't like them because they're not men, and women don't like them because they're weak and not a man. If you are a pregnant mother or expect to be one in the future, for your son's sake, don't drink water from soft-plastic bottles.

Next, is water that comes in hard-plastic bottles, the five-gallon drums that water-bottling companies use. Hopefully they are using BPA-free plastic containers, call them and ask. Hard plastics are generally better than soft plastics, but the BPA baby bottles that were banned were hard plastic, and some of those blue five-gallon water jugs have a #7 on the bottom which is known for containing BPA. If you buy a BPA-free hard-plastic five-gallon container that's never had water in it, fill it to the brim with water and let it sit 24 hours and then discard the water, and do this every day for a week before you begin using it for drinking. I subscribed to *Men's Health* magazine and my issue would arrive in a sealed plastic bag. When I opened the bag, wow! Paint and printing chemicals flooded my nose. From then on, I would open it outside and let it air out for a week before handling it and bringing it inside. Dry-cleaned clothes are the same thing, you should remove the plastic bag outside and let your clothes off-gas outside before bringing them into your house. So, the hard-plastic five-gallon containers used by the bottling companies may be fine if it's BPA-free, unless your bottle is a brand-new plastic bottle that arrived at the bottling company and the plastic is still fresh and you are the first customer to drink from it. But as far as the water itself is concerned, it is typically delicious, tasty, fresh mountain spring water, and as stated earlier, the pH is usually pretty close to what water should be, 7. This water also has the added benefits of having trace minerals from the mountain runoff, like you hear of those cultures that live in remote areas of the world and live to be 100 years old drinking pure clean mineral water. I've never heard them say what the pH is of that water that these cultures drink, but undoubtedly it is 7 or higher due to its pure source and its rich mineral content.

Medium plastics, those that aren't soft and flexible but aren't hard like the five-gallon drums, I put these semi-hard plastics in the same category as soft plastics. Apparently the #2 HDPE plastics don't leach, but they are still slightly soft. Use glass and then you don't have to worry about it. Even if it says BPA-free, there are other plastic chemicals that you don't need to be exposing yourself to.

Stainless-steel drinking cups are out as well. They say stainless steel doesn't leach but why use metal when you can use glass. Plus, metal is never 100% pure metal. A 14-karat gold-necklace is only 58% gold. The rest is nickel, silver, and who knows what else, mercury, cadmium, lead? Some people say that if the stainless-steel cup has a 0.18 on the bottom then it's safe to use with acid beverages like colas and coffee. Just use glass.

Next, is tap water from your local municipality. Although many people drink this water, unfiltered, straight from the tap, a steady diet of this type of water may cause future health problems for you. All municipal drinking-water is chlorinated, (bleached), to kill coliforms, (bacteria), and viruses. The chlorine concentration may even be sufficient to kill amoebas, worms and flukes, but I know for a fact that parasite EGGS are not killed with low concentrations of chlorine. Worm eggs are like spores, they are walled-off, and this wall protects the life-form from being destroyed. It's the organism's survival mechanism. So, do you have parasite eggs coming out of your faucet, not likely, but it does happen and it is possible. But worse than biology is, CHEMISTRY. The chemicals that inadvertently get into the water supply. I knew of a doctor's wife who had a chemistry degree, and she had health issues that couldn't be pinpointed. In the process of trouble-shooting her life for the source of the problem, she determined that it was due to the arsenic in her tap water. She had a reverse-osmosis system installed at the entry point to their home and her symptoms faded away. I've drank tap water before, but I think you are taking a bit of a gamble by drinking it every day long term. I read where certain of the soldiers in the Vietnam War had garden hose like veins and arteries when they came home. It is theorized that the chlorine tablets used to purify their drinking-water caused their endothelial linings to inflame and the body's response was to thicken them. I have personally drawn blood from people with "garden-hose" veins. You have to pin down the part of the vein that you are going to draw blood from and then jab the needle in, otherwise, you can't get the needle to go through the vein because their veins are just so thick and hard. I believe that chlorine can do this, in a short period of time, in the case of the soldiers and the chlorine tablets, or over a longer period of time, in the case of chlorinated drinking-water.

Charcoal-filtered tap water is not ideal either. People don't change the filters often enough, and if they do, all it takes is a blast of contaminants coming through your faucet and now your brand-new filter is contaminated. That's not likely to happen too often, but it can and it does. Remember the doctor's wife and the trace amounts of arsenic exposure that was affecting her. If you feel signs of lethargy, maybe it's just your drinking-water.

Distilled water is usually recommended in the same sentence as Reverse Osmosis water, but they are not the same. Both types of water are 100% pure H_2O water molecules, but distilled water is heated and reverse osmosis is not. Water distillers heat the water to create water vapor, steam, then the water vapor is captured through condensation and collected for drinking. It is pure water, but it's cooked. With reverse osmosis, tap water is forced through a filter with tiny pores that allows only water molecules to pass through. The filtered water is collected, and the brine water goes down the drain. It's a bit wasteful, but it does create pure water. Both distilled water and reverse-osmosis water lack trace minerals, so I supplement with minerals, calcium, magnesium, zinc, copper, iron, iodine, chromium, selenium, boron, manganese, and MSM (Methyl Sulfonyl Methane, organic sulfur).

Some supermarkets have reverse-osmosis machines in their stores and you can bring your own glass gallon jugs and fill up for only $0.39 per gallon or four gallons for $1.56. This is a good option. The outdoor reverse-osmosis machines aren't too clean looking so I would stay away from them. You simply can't get around the street dust, air pollution, and who knows if someone has purposely contaminated them as a bad prank. The in-store machines are clean and maintained and the store is liable for obvious contamination, so look for in-store reverse osmosis, or buy a reverse-osmosis filter and attach it to your kitchen faucet. The one I have is the Aquawizard 2, (800) 872-8081. It costs about $200, but $46 is for the TDS meter, Total Dissolved Solutes meter. My unfiltered tap water has a total dissolved solutes of about 220. With the filter, it drops it down to about 7.

Next! The containers!

CHAPTER 7

THE CONTAINERS

Along with the ABC Water, you'll need a storage container and a drinking container. The storage container is a one-gallon glass bottle, and the drinking container is a one-liter 32oz glass jar with screw cap and a glass straw. If you still use plastic, consider this. Just imagine how many millions of plastic water bottles are produced and disposed of year after year after year. Before the 1990s, before bottled water made its big entrance into the market, I never saw a plastic water bottle at the beach or in the ocean, or in rivers and lakes. I really believe that the plastic-water-bottle companies and the people behind the huge shift in the public's thinking, that plastic bottled water is better than tap water, are the same people or companies that told us that, "Margarine is better than butter and good for your heart," when in fact the world has now been told that Trans Fat is the most toxic fat in the grocery store. So the earth isn't flat after all. Hm. Now they are making margarine Fully hydrogenated instead of Partially hydrogenated, well, running hydrogen gas through a liquid oil using nickel probes is simply adulteration.

So go green with glass! You purchase it once, you don't throw anything in the trash, and you don't leave behind a carbon footprint. Here's something else I noticed when I switched from plastic to glass, my food and drink tastes cleaner! My most recent switch was from a plastic straw to a glass straw. I resisted at first because of the price, $9 per straw, but what a difference. Most people have never used a glass straw so the thought that their beverage will taste better hasn't crossed their minds. I am sold. Plus, no more breaking of my plastic straw when I'm hauling it from point A to point B, from the house to the car et cetera. To break the glass straw you would have to drop it on the floor as the company has designed it to be quite breakproof. This is true for the one-gallon bottle and the one-quart jar as well, the glass is very strong.

For the glass gallon bottles, go to Container And Packaging, www.containerandpackaging.com (800) 473-4144. Type "glass gallon" in the search-box and you will see one-gallon glass jugs, item G002, four per case for $15.40. They will charge you $10 for a small order of less-than $50 so why not buy the master case of 16 bottles for $50.40 and give three cases away as gifts. They don't come with caps so you will need to order item L088, 38-400 Black Phenolic Lid with Polycone Liner. I chose this cap because of the airtight seal the cone liner makes, allowing you to store the ABC Water on its side without it leaking. Each cap is $0.63, so you'll need to order 4 or 16, and a couple of extras in case you lose one. The bottle with cap is 11⅞ inches tall so you will need 12 inches of height space in your refrigerator. If you decide to store it on its side, you will need 6½ inches of height space.

Alternatively, you can purchase a gallon of organic apple juice from your local healthfood store. After drinking the juice, scrub off the label and you'll have a one-gallon glass bottle, however, the aluminum cap won't allow you to store it on its side.

I have a Kenmore Freezerless Refrigerator 16.7cu.ft, model #60722, that I purchased at Sears.com for less-than $500, currently selling for $552. The fourth shelf fits 8 gallons, 2 rows of 4, perfectly. If you haven't switched over to a freezerless refrigerator, I recommend you do so. Eating homemade food is key to maintaining weight and good health, and the freezerless refrigerator, with its plenty of space and shelves, makes meal making and food prep extremely user-friendly. You can add plastic trays to the shelves, and acrylic cube containers in the door shelves, and label them with your Dymo label maker. Your food items and meals are organized, tidy, easy to access, and you can see everything at a glance. Thank you Kenmore, or whoever it was that came up with the idea for an all-refrigeration refrigerator!

The second half of this publication, the Number Crunch Diet™, is based on preparing your own Pre-Counted Meals™, which allows you to keep track of your calories by simply counting the number of meals you eat each day. So if you have this freezerless refrigerator, you can place all your pre-made breakfast meals on the first shelf, all your lunch meals on the second shelf, all your dinner meals on the third shelf, your ABC Water goes on the fourth shelf, and on the bottom shelf you can place miscellaneous items and snacks. It's perfect, in that it makes eating and meal making fast, fun, and efficient. After all, you don't want to get bogged down in the kitchen, when the purpose of your refrigerator is to store the energy and nutrition you need to live your life.

The glass one-quart container-jar is available at Container And Packaging, but let's go to SKS Science to purchase them, as they have other sizes you'll want to think about buying, such as, 16oz 12oz 8oz 6oz 4oz 2oz and 1oz. The web address is www.sks-bottle.com. Many many people over the years have asked me, "Where did you get that container?" Well, here it is world. My secret website where I purchased all of my glass food containers! No more plastic. I can heat my food in the microwave directly from these glass containers. The clarity and quality is excellent so you can see what's inside. The white caps add a clean touch to the look. But here's the best feature. Food lasts 2-3 times LONGER!

Yes, by using glass containers, filling them to the top, and then using a screw cap to seal it, it's almost as though you are canning or preserving your food. If you fill the container full to the brim, which most of my meal recipes are, then screw on the cap and refrigerate, your meals can last 10-14 days without spoiling! This is amazing! My sole purpose was to get away from eating out of plastic and switch to cleaner nontoxic glass. But the bonus was, double and triple the normal expiration dates of my meals.

So as we shop for the one-quart container, think seriously about purchasing a case of all the other sizes. You see, the less air the better, when storing a meal. So if you have one cup of food, you will want to store it in an 8oz container. If you store one cup of food in a 16oz container then the container contains one cup of food and one cup of air. This air, with its 21% oxygen content, is going to make your food spoil. Then you have to throw it away, or worse, you don't realize it's starting to spoil, and you eat it and end up with digestive problems. It will cost you some money in the beginning, but you have to buy food containers anyway if you are going to make and store food. Give your old containers away or take them to the Goodwill, and switch to glass.

Someone was showing me a Tupperware catalogue once and the first thing I noticed were the high prices. The containers were strong plastic containers with tight-fitting lids, but they weren't clear glass, so you can't see what's inside, the lids aren't as user-friendly as screw caps, and glass doesn't leach, not even when heated, whereas you can't say that about plastic. If you use something every day, then it's worth the financial investment to spend the money.

You will also want to go to Walmart, if you haven't already done so, and purchase the Pyrex glass bowls and rectangles with the red lids. Before they started selling these glass food containers, they sold Rubbermaid plastic food containers. So thank you Walmart for replacing your plastic food containers with glass, and thank you Pyrex for making glass food containers. KEEP IT UP! We want more sizes and shapes! And make the bowls with screw caps instead of lids for longer food-expiration dates!

Okay! The moment you've all been waiting for! Glass food containers with screw caps! You saw it here first! My secret website…www.sks-bottle.com. Click on "Glass Containers" on the left. Then click "Glass Jars" from the dropdown menu. Click on the "Clear Glass Jars with White Lined Caps" image. Scroll down a bit to see the "Glass Jars Only Bulk" and there you have all the sizes that I have purchased. I suggest starting with 24 of each size, starting with one case of 2oz, one case of 4oz, one case of 6oz, one case of 8oz, two cases of 12oz, and two cases of 16oz, and two cases of 32oz. You will be surprised when you realize how handy they are for many things besides food. Now, these bulk jars don't come with caps, so you'll need to click on the cap image to the right under "add-ons" to see a list of available caps. I recommend the UN-lined caps, the "white polypro ribbed unlined" caps, or you could go with the "white smooth plastic unlined" caps. Originally I bought the jars with the caps included, as shown at the top of the page, but over time, the edges of the liners loosened, and moisture got underneath and mold grew.   So learn from my mistake and go with the unlined caps. The caps come in all sizes to fit the sizes of the jars, and you will end up with a lot of extra caps as there are 144 caps in a bag, but the bulk jars are 40% less in price than the jars with lined caps. You might try calling them and ask them if you can substitute unlined caps for the lined caps and see what they say. The other option is to go back to Container & Packaging and buy the caps there, as they sell the same caps and you can purchase any number that you like, but plan your order in advance so that you purchase a minimum of $50, avoiding the $10 small-order fee.

So there you have it. You can review your options and decide. If you spend $250 or more at sks-bottle.com the shipping is free, otherwise, the shipping can cost more than your order because glass is heavy. So spend some time thinking about it and figure out the best strategy for you. My first choice would be to buy $250 of containers from sks-bottle.com and choose the jars with caps, but ask them if they will substitute unlined caps for the lined caps, this way you get free shipping, and $250 will be sufficient to stock your kitchen cupboards with glass food containers in all sizes that you will use over-and-over every day of your life.

In addition to the 2 4 6 8 12 16 and 32 ounce jars, I also purchased a case of the 1oz with lined caps, and these liners seem to stay snug around the edges, because the caps are small. It's the 2oz lined caps and larger where the liners loosen and come off over time. Again, you might think you don't need all these sizes, but you don't want to put half a cup of food in an 8oz container and have 4oz of air on top. You want to have different sizes to fit your needs.

So for your ABC Water™, you will be using the 32oz glass jar with unlined cap. Having a few extra caps is a good idea, because if you do drop the jar, the jar might not break, but the cap will, so then you end up with a jar and no cap. This is where C&P comes in handy, as you can buy one or five or any number that you want.

Now you're going to drill a hole in your lid for the straw. If you are going to use a plastic straw, I used the ones from Smart & Final grocery and restaurant-supply store. I bought a box of 500 red jumbo straws, 10.25 inches long, for about $5. If I used one a day, then that's about a 15 month supply. Use a ¼-inch drill bit to drill a hole in the center of your lid. Make 3-4 lids so that if one or two are in the dishwasher, you have some clean ones available. Then, smooth out the edges of the hole with a cloth, and you're done. Since the jar is 6.75 inches tall, your straw will be sticking up 3.5 inches, and you may find you want to go with a shorter straw so they don't break as easily. Or you can, should, use a glass straw.

I bought mine at Lassen's Health Foods, and it's made by Foods Alive, www.foodsalive.com. Click on "products", then click "glass straw" from the dropdown menu. Choose the 8-inch glass drinking straw as this will leave you with about 1.5 inches sticking up above the lid. Their website states, "environmentally friendly and extremely elegant". Ever noticed how in the workplace people try to pretend like they have money, or that they come from a family with money, more money than you have? Well, walk into your job with a $9 straw and see how many heads turn. If your coworkers judge you by the labels on your clothes, then show up with a glass water bottle and glass straw and see who has more class. And more smarts.

Underneath the "Add To Cart" it reads, "When you use a glass straw, you reduce the number of straws that end up in our landfills, and avoid consuming the toxins that plastic straws can leach into your drinks."

Did you know that crystal contains lead, or it used to, and that the higher the lead content the more expensive the crystal is because it gives a louder "pinging" sound when you tap it? At one store here in town, they used to have a "Proposition 65" warning sign on the shelf with the crystal stating that it contained lead, known to the State of California to cause cancer and birth defects. When I told this to someone, she said, "Oh yeah, and the more lead the better the crystal." Anyway, Foods Alive glass straws are 100% made in the USA and free from heavy metals like lead, mercury, and cadmium, so support this company, they are doing something cutting-edge and good for people.

Drilling the hole for the glass straw, use a ⅜-inch drill bit, placing the point of the drill bit directly in the center of the lid, then smooth out the hole with a cloth.

When I came up with this idea, a product really, I wanted to patent it. There are people on TV saying that you should be drinking out of glass but it's hard to find and they themselves don't know where to find glass drinking containers. Well, here it is. Go to sks-bottle and place a $250 order and include the other sizes in your order and get started on your way to glass. I wouldn't be surprised, and heartbroken, if somebody takes the information in this chapter and starts selling 32oz glass jars with a screw-cap lid and hole in it with a glass straw, and begins advertising them on "As Seen On TV".

That said, I hereby name the above, the ABC Water Glass Beverage Container™.

CHAPTER 8

RECAP

Let's take a few minutes to recap what's been covered so far.

1. These statements are my own personal experiences. The reader must decide what's best for him or herself.

2. The companies mentioned are completely unaware that I am promoting them, and I do so only because I personally like their products.

3. Top-of-the-list, number one thing that I consider to be of prime health importance is, stocking up your alkaline stores and keeping them stocked. Your first choice for doing this is, to cut back on dietary animal foods and junk foods, and add in more fresh fruits and vegetables, preferably organic and whatever's in season. Additionally, increase dietary alkalinity to compensate for hard physical exercise and mental stress; mental stress, anger, anguish, worry, 24-hour turmoil, being the worst of all acid-producers.

4. Since a vegan diet is not an option for many of us, myself included, the next thing you can do is to supplement with bicarbonate. But before you do so, you need to determine your current alkaline status to see where you're at.

5. One quart of ABC Water a day contains one-fourth capsule of vitamin B complex, so you are not in any danger of taking too

much, as this works out to less-than two capsules a week, or 7.5 capsules a month, or one bottle of 100 capsules per year. On the contrary, this is what you should be doing so that you're never without B vitamins.

6. One quart of ABC Water contains about 570mg of vitamin C, which is significantly higher than the RDA, but we all know that the RDAs are really the minimums needed to prevent disease. You need more for optimum health as vitamin C is responsible for DAMAGE CONTROL. I have a multivitamin mineral supplement that says to take two tablets per day, providing 1000mg per day of vitamin C. So, 500 or 570mg taken gradually throughout your 16-hour day is not dangerous, but rather, it's giving your bloodstream a steady supply of the antioxidant power it needs. Both B and C are water-soluble so any excess, if there is any, will be washed out into the urine.

7. Your first choice for drinking-water is to make your own reverse-osmosis water at home from tap water and collecting it into glass gallon bottles. The next best option, is to take your glass gallon bottles to the supermarket and fill them at their in-store reverse-osmosis machine. The third best option is to drink tap water, or filtered tap water, or buy five-gallon jugs of water from a bottling company. Water that comes in soft-plastic containers is not an option.

8. If you are looking to buy a refrigerator, go freezerless, or add a second refrigerator, freezerless, to your home. Ample refrigeration space is essential for someone who makes their own meals, Number Crunch Diet™ style.

9. If you have plastic food containers and you can afford it, toss them in the trash. Plastic food containers was just a bad idea from the get-go, especially if you are putting them in the microwave. Switch to glass food containers, Pyrex, SKS, C&P.

10. Show the world how classy you are and how informed and cutting-edge you are by drinking your beverage from a glass

container using a $9 glass straw.

Chapter Endnote

According to the rules of grammar, an exclamation mark (!) is used at the end of a sentence only. But what if you want to exclaim a word within a sentence? The dictionary example of the word "amazing" was, "She makes the most amazing cakes." Yawn. So, just to give you a heads-up, you will see "!" punctuation as part of the word within a sentence. Certain words have to be written with energy!, or even ENERGY!!, just like how you would say them.

Also, you may have noticed that when there's a quotation within a sentence, that I place the comma on the outside of the quotation mark. Many writers and grammarians say you should place the comma inside the quotation. However, this gives the impression that the comma is part of the quotation. I keep my quotations "clean", and place the comma on the outside. Sorry grammarians.

Lastly, to calculate the percent of something, take the amount number, divide it by the total number, then multiply by 100. For example, if I have 26 of something, and 35 total, then $26 \div 35 = 0.74$, times $100 = 74\%$.

CHAPTER 9

pH

Perhaps you remember from school that pH is a measure of acid and base and that water is neutral with a pH of 7. Less-than 7 is acidic, greater-than 7 is alkaline. Our blood needs to be slightly alkaline at pH 7.4. People that arrive at the emergency room having a blood pH of 6.8 are typically dead on arrival.

The H in pH stands for hydrogen ion, H+. It's an acid. You know that your stomach secretes HCl or hydrochloric acid. The H part is the acid. In the stomach, acid is a good thing, you want this, because acid is needed to break down the protein in your meal into amino acids. A lot of people have stomach acid problems, not enough acid, too much acid, or ulcers due to acid secretion when there's nothing in the stomach. This is a body gone wrong. To pinpoint the root cause of your problem could be impossible. A healthy body shouldn't have stomach acid problems. It could be that if you just balance your acid alkaline status all your symptoms might go away. Rather than treat the problem, fix your health status, and the problem goes away as a byproduct of having good health.

Some people believe that your urine pH should be acidic, I say not so, unless you're fighting a urinary tract infection, in which case, acidifying the urine can help to reduce certain kinds of bacteria. But a normal healthy body should have a balance of acid neutralization going on in the body, and this gets reflected in the urine. Quite simply, if you have enough alkaline reserves in your body, your urine should be being excreted at just a little below the pH of the blood, at about 7. If you don't have enough alkaline reserves, then your body is going to hold on to any and all alkaline that you have and your urine is going to be excreted as an acid, pH 5 or 6.

I was working in the microbiology department of a lab one day and the microbiology supervisor said to me, "Don't work up that yeast, few yeast is normal." So I went over to the director and said, "Director, few yeast, it that normal?" I never got an answer. Here's my point. Just because something is COMMOM, it doesn't make it NORMAL.

A similar thing happened in the chemistry department. Many of the alkaline phosphatase (ALP) results in this particular batch of blood samples were high, 100-200. I was told, "It's just normal for this patient population." In some instances yes, but the truth is, alkaline phosphatase was being released from their bones because they drink colas, colas being high in phosphoric acid, and the phosphates pull calcium out of the body. To make matters worse, colas are acidic, and an acid environment dissolves bone, and teeth.

So with regard to urine pH, just because it's COMMON to have a urine pH of 5, that doesn't make it NORMAL. I'd like someone to test the pH of a group of healthy people who have been strict vegetarians all their lives. And not people in their 50s or 60s who may already be alkaline deficient from aging, but healthy young vegetarians. These people will have a urine pH of 7.

So our goal is, to have the internal environment of a young healthy vegetarian, while living a stressful lifestyle, eating animal protein, few fruits and vegetables, and working out 3x a week in our attempt to get in shape and look fit. That's a tall order. Fortunately we have the ABC Water™. A way to supplement with alkalinity to compensate for our high-acid low-alkaline lifestyles.

Now, the opposite of acid is alkaline, and as stated, your blood, that LIFE FORCE FLUID that bathes your organs and tissues, needs to be slightly alkaline, 7.4. Think of acid and base as a business bank account, in one column you have things that add, in the other column you have things that subtract. You need to keep your bank account a little on the plus side. Too many subtractions without enough additions can result in the closure of your business.

Picture a balance scale, the Lady of Justice holds one in her left hand. When the two sides of the scale are level, that's pH 7, neutral. If the scale tips to the left, that's acidic, 6 5 4 3 2 1. If the scale tips to the right, that's a lack of acid, or alkaline, 8 9 10 11 12.

The pH scale goes from 0 to 14, with 7 being the middle of the scale and pH neutral. If I had made this scale, I might have chosen neutral as zero, and +1 +2 +3 +4 +5 as alkaline, and -1 -2 -3 -4 -5 as acidic. Referring back to the bank account again, if you have more deposits, you have more credits, more money, and if you have more withdrawals, you have more debits, more debt, more deficit, deficiency. Alkaline and acid can be looked at in the same way, and you can flip the words back-and-forth, high alkalinity means low acidity, and high acidity means low alkalinity. Lots of credits means low debt, lots of debits means low money in your bank account. You want your body to have a sufficient account balance of alkalinity. NSF, no sufficient funds, as the bank would say, is not healthy.

With regard to your blood, the range is tight, 7.35 to 7.45, with the middle being 7.4. If it drops to below 7.2, that's considered critical. If it drops to below 7.0, as they say in the hospital world, you're "circling-the-drain". And if it continues dropping and stays there, you're "EXP" expired. Your tissues are fried, boiled in acid. Many many people who die in a hospital die in this acidotic state of the blood. Now one might argue, "they died of a heart attack". A lot of things in life are, "Which came first, the chicken or the egg?" Did the heart explode on its own resulting in the acid, or was the person in an already acidic state that caused the heart to explode? I'll let you think about that.

The counterpart to H+ acid is bicarbonate, HCO_3-. Baking soda is one sodium and one bicarbonate, $NaHCO_3$. Think of bicarbonate as the hero. It comes in and mops up the acid, thereby keeping your blood pH from dropping.

An alkaline diet, the vegan vegetarian diet, is the best way to keep the acid from becoming a problem. Unfortunately, most of us simply aren't willing to give up animal products and eat a plant-based diet. On top of that, fruit has sugar and sugar raises insulin and insulin takes the excess sugar and stores it as fat. With two-thirds of the population being overweight, sugar is now regarded as evil and the cause of all health problems. This is partly true. But this has led to people being afraid of eating fruit. And if you want to drop fat you really do have to cut out sugar. So now, your dietary consumption of vegetables takes on the brunt of the job of mopping up the acid. But how many vegetables are we getting each and every day? Add to this the high pressure that many people are living with 24-hours-a-day 7-days-a-week that's keeping them in a constant state of mental acidosis, aka, anxiety.

Is it any wonder so many people are sick? There simply isn't enough alkalinity in our lives to mop up the acid of our modern lifestyles. The scales are tipped to the wrong side.

But there is a workaround solution to acidosis for those who aren't vegetarians or who eat few if any fruits and vegetables. You can supplement with bicarbonate. But you have to do it sensibly and responsibly. You have to first determine your current alkaline status, if you are low, then you have to stock up your stores, then determine how much you need to maintain. It's similar to going on a diet. You first determine where you're at, then you take action to get to where you want to be, then you maintain. And just like dieting, you have to know what you're doing. With dieting, you want to track your calories, with alkalinity, you want to track your urine pH.

CHAPTER 10

Where you at?

There may be other ways to determine your alkaline status, and you are free to look them up and try them. No, I haven't forgotten about saliva pH, and pH challenge tests, I'm just going to keep it simple. This chapter will cover the way I determined my starting-point alkaline status. I created it, and I like it. It's simple and it makes sense. So here we go.

Once you get your pH paper purchased and set up, see next chapter, before you begin drinking the ABC Water, you will test the pH of all of your urinations for one week.

Label a binder and hole punch some cardstock, 20 lb paper gets to be too flimsy and messy. You can purchase 110 lb white cardstock 250 sheets at Walmart for about $6.50. You want to be able to clearly read what numbers you've written down, and be able to look back and see patterns. You want to get familiar with your urine-pH numbers.

Obtain three pens, one green, one blue, and one red, and a clipboard.

Using a ruler or spreadsheet software, make a chart with Mon Tue Wed Thu Fri Sat Sun along the left side, and times of the day along the top. If you get up at 06:00 and go to bed at 22:00, then make 16 vertical columns for the times, 6 7 8 9 10 11 Noon, etc., across the top. Okay, you have a grid, a weekly chart.

The most telling urine-pH number is the one when you first get up.
Never miss testing this one.

Be diligent about this week, take your pH-paper strips with you and
record the numbers on a piece of paper and transcribe those
numbers onto your chart when you get home. You don't have to be
super accurate with the times, but it will help you to see patterns
when the week is completed.   If you miss some measurements
because you forgot, it will make it harder to see patterns at the end
of the week, in which case, if you miss testing too many of your
urinations, start over and be more diligent.

Record on your chart in red any pH that's a 5 something, so 5, 5.5.
Record in blue any pH that's a 6 something, 6, 6.2, 6.4, 6.6, 6.8.
Record in green any 7, 7.2, 7.4. You likely won't see 7.2 or 7.4 or
higher unless you have a urinary-tract infection with *Proteus*, or
you've eaten a lot of fruits and vegetables and no meat, or you have
a kidney defect, or your alkaline stores are empty and you're
making ammonia, in which case, all of these, except the fruits-and-
vegetables person, should seek professional medical care, as a
selfcare book is not the way you should proceed, although I believe
your bodies are toxic with acid, especially the ammonia person.

At the end of the week, add up the total number of reds, the total
number of blues, the total number of greens, and the total number
of measurements. When I did this, I had about five urinations a
day and so I had 35 total measurements. Refer to the definitions
below to find your score.

10	All of your readings were red	HIGHLY ACIDIC
9	90% of your readings were red	Highly Acidic
8	80% of your readings were red	highly acidic
7	70% of your readings were red	Mod to Highly Acidic
6	60% of your readings were red	mod to highly acidic
5	50% of your readings were red	Moderately Acidic
4	40% of your readings were red	moderately acidic

3   30% of your readings were red   Some Acid
2   20% of your readings were red   Slightly Acidic
1   10% of your readings were red   Occasionally Acidic
0   No reds. Rarely Acidic. This person is likely a vegetarian.

The goal is to have all of your urinations be 7. Not less-than 7 and definitely not less-than 6.

If when you start the ABC Water you get a 7.2, then no more ABC Water for the remainder of the day. If you should get a 7.4, then no more ABC Water for 24 hours or longer.

Your target is 7. Not 7.2 not 7.4, but 7 exactly. You don't want to overshoot.

When I did this, my score was about a 7.5 with 75% of my numbers being 5s, and the remaining 25% being 6s, with no 7s.

I started with a ½t per day of baking soda with almost no change in urine pH. I was alkaline depleted and my body sucked it up.

So I doubled it to 1t per day, and I started to see half 6s and half 5s.

So I doubled it again to 2t per day, sipping the water GRADUALLY throughout the day, not all at one time. Now I was starting to see some 7s, but no 7.2s. However, my first morning pH would be 5, and I had fatigue. I was determined to get rid of all the 5s, and eventually, at the end of the third week, I did. That's when I encountered a slight frontal headache, and when I checked my urine pH it was 7.4. I overshot, but that's okay, by my next urination it was 7 and then 6.4.

So for me, it took three weeks to stock up my stores at about 2t per day. Then I cut back to 1t per day.

But it doesn't stop there. I discovered that hard exercise increases my need for alkalinity due to the fact that hard physical work, that makes your muscles sore the next day, produces acid. So that's when I amended my 1t-a-day rule to include an additional ½t on days that I do 30 minutes of hard physical exercise, or 60 minutes of moderate physical exercise.

Since then, I have also added on a second amendment, and that is, an additional ½t if the night before I didn't sleep well because something was on my mind, "worry". Now I don't think of myself as someone who worries, but it can simply be anything that bothered you during the day that you failed to let go of, and you didn't notice that it was still stuck to you, and you went to bed, and boom! You wake up the next morning feeling like you were in a brawl the night before. Watching the news before bed can do the same thing. Instead of a restful-night's sleep, you're affected by what's going on in the news and that plays out during your sleep. This is why mental stress is so bad. It drains your alkaline batteries.

So I have my one quart of ABC Water per day, (1t bicarbonate), with my two amendments, one for exercise, one for stress.

I hope you are excited to find out your personal acid alkaline status and personal needs for supplementation. Take the time to do it properly and responsibly and diligently so you can see the changes, see patterns, and get to know your body when your urine pH is 5, 6 and 7. Try to spot alkaline tides, times of the day when your urine pH just goes up for no apparent reason. Science claims it happens after a meal, due to the loss of acid that occurs when HCl is secreted into the stomach, others say it's at 10:00 and 22:00. I don't think those are hard-and-fast rules, there's too much variability amongst people's diets, biorhythms, schedules, activity levels, and thinking. Remember, some strong upset can change your entire body's physiology in minutes. And be alert and on the lookout for that day when, all of a sudden your alkaline stores are stocked up and you don't need as much. At that point you switch from Stocking-Up Mode, to Maintenance Mode, with the goal of maintaining your urine pH at exactly 7.0.

CHAPTER 11

pH Paper

To test and track your urine pH, you will need pH paper. Think of all the things in life that people check, the fluids in their vehicle, coolant level, oil color and level, tire pressure, your bank account, credit-card statement, retirement account, your weight, blood pressure, and on and on. Checking the status of the internal environment of your body, the "vehicle" that makes or breaks your life, should be of paramount importance to you.

I purchased pH paper from www.microessentiallab.com Micro Essential Lab (718) 338-3618. Their products are also available on Amazon.com, but you may not be able to find the exact rolls. Click on "pH paper" on the left. Click "Jumbo pH Paper" on the left. There you will see five products to choose from, all "Jumbo" rolls, meaning that they are a **1/2** inch wide and **50** feet long.

I purchased 5 rolls of HJ-613, pH range 0-13, and I also purchased 5 rolls of HJ-633, pH range 6-8. So, 5 rolls of general and 5 rolls of specific. Now you might think this is far too much, but the paper lasts forever, providing you store it properly, and in the beginning you will be trying to get to know your body's acid alkaline status and how it's affected, so you will be using about ten test strips per day. Another reason for purchasing what may seem like a lifetime supply, is that, one day government might decide that pH paper is illegal and pull it off the market. I used to buy Red Devil lye crystals at the supermarket to make my own soap, but they pulled it off the supermarket shelves and now lye is only available in liquid bottles, which requires using half a bottle to clear a slow drain, whereas one spoonful of the lye crystals worked wonders. So, who knows what will be considered "dangerous" in the future, they may even take baking soda off the shelves if too many people begin ridding themselves of acidosis and gaining their health back by alkalizing their internal environment. What would happen if an industry began to see a gradual steady loss of its customers because its clients found their own solution?

The 0-13 paper allows you to read your urine pH at 5, 6, 7, and 8, whole number readings. You won't see urine readings of 4 and 9, as your body can only make urine in the range of 4.5 to 8. Now it is possible to see a urine pH of 9, which can occur if you have a UTI and the bacteria is *Proteus*, in which case you will want to acidify your urine pH by drinking cranberry juice and see a doctor for antibiotics and a urine culture. But this is not a medical book for medical problems, it's a selfcare book for optimum health. But for most people, you will see urine readings of 5, 6, and 7. Now if the color of your paper is halfway between 5 and 6, you can say it's 5.5. Or if the color is not quite as green as the green for the 7, you can say it's 6.8. This is why I also bought the 6-8 paper, for more specific readings.

The 6-8 paper gives readings at 6, 6.4, 6.8, 7, 7.2, 7.6, and 8. If you get a reading of 6, you will want to also use the 0-13 paper because your reading may be 5, 5.5, or 6. In other words, if the paper reads 6, it might be 6, or it might be less-than 6, you don't know. I really make sure to avoid letting my urine become 5. I definitely notice that drained feeling when my urine pH is 5. As stated previously, your goal is to get your urine pH up to 7 and keep it there. Picture yourself driving onto the freeway, accelerating to 70 mph, and then locking in with the cruise-control button. If you drop down to 6, or 60 mph, you feel like you're slowing down. If you drop down to 5, or 50 mph, you really notice you've slowed down. If you accidentally overshoot and find yourself at 72 or 74 mph, or pH 7.2 or 7.4, then back off the bicarb gas pedal, and slow it down to 7.

As with the 0-13 paper, you can read between the readings with the 6-8 paper. So if the color is halfway between 6 and 6.4, you can record 6.2, or if the color is halfway between 6.4 and 6.8, you can record 6.6. This paper allows you to see how much below 7 you have fallen. If your reading is 6.8, no worries, you're not far from the ideal 7. If your reading is 6.2, well, as with my situation, I would drink 8 sips of ABC Water to get back up to pH 7. If I didn't, then my next urine pH 3-4 hours later would be 5.5 or 5.

So start by using both the 0-13 paper and the 6-8 paper. Later on, when you are good at keeping your urine at 7, then just use the 6-8 paper, remembering to retest with the 0-13 paper if you get a 6, to confirm that it's really a 6, and not a 5 or a 5.5.

The rolls are $10.73 each and the minimum purchase is 5 rolls, so that's $53.65 for the 0-13 paper, and $53.65 for the 6-8 paper, plus shipping, so about $120. Now that might seem like a lot, but it will last you five or more years for one person, in which case it works out to $2 a month to monitor and track your body's acid alkaline status. Later on when you figure out your own body's needs for additional alkalinity, then you can do as I have done and just check your first morning pH only, and spot-check whenever you feel your energy crashing. This may mean that your pH paper will last you ten years, costing $1 per month.

You may find pH paper sold elsewhere, amazon.com sells single rolls, but you may not be able to find these exact rolls, and then you may not be saving money in the long run. Plus, if you keep running out of paper every few months because you bought the 15-foot rolls, you will eventually phase out this beneficial lifestyle habit, or you may decide you just don't want to keep spending $15 every few months and drop the idea altogether. I want to help you succeed with this, because I know how important internal pH is to body health. Also, you don't know if the resellers on amazon have stored the paper properly, with regard to temperature, light, and humidity, it may be okay or it may not be okay. This is why it's better to do it right and buy the 50-foot jumbo rolls direct from the manufacturer, microessentiallab.com.

When the rolls arrive, take 4 rolls of the 0-13 paper and remove them from their plastic cases, don't remove the foil wrapper, and place the color charts aside. Using a vacuum sealer, seal each roll in its own vacuum-seal bag. Use a pen to label them "pH 0-13" and today's date. Do the same with the 4 rolls of the 6-8 paper, labeling them "pH 6-8" and the date. Place the 8 rolls, 4 and 4, in a brown-paper bag and write "pH paper" on it. Store it in a dry place at room temperature.

Next, you will need to find two containers for your pH-paper strips. Deli containers work perfectly for this. See if your supermarket deli will sell you two 8oz clear-plastic deli containers with lids. I purchased a bag of 50 containers and 50 lids at Smart & Final supermarket and restaurant-supply store. The containers come in handy for other things, which for me, is to store my homemade bars of soap. For my pH paper, I actually use the 6oz deli container as it's slightly shorter and I like it better. For those of you who don't know what a deli container is, picture a 16oz one-pound plastic container of cottage cheese. Now imagine that it's half as tall, 8oz, or a bit shorter, 6oz, and that the plastic is clear. I suppose you could buy an 8oz container of hummus dip and remove the labels and wash it clean. Okay, now take your 0-13 color chart and place it upside down on the inside of the lid, taping it on all four sides. Now place the lid on the container and voila, you can see the color chart. By placing the color chart on the inside of the lid, you will protect the chart from water and moisture damage ensuring that the chart will last. By using a clear-plastic container, the chart colors are clearly visible. Do the same thing with the 6-8 color chart and deli-container lid. When you are done, you will have two deli containers, one with the 0-13 color chart on the lid, and the other with the 6-8 color chart on the lid. Now you're ready to fill them up with paper strips.

The nice thing about the Smart & Final deli containers is that they are lightweight, easy to open and close, and the lid creates an airtight seal, and they don't wear out. Amazing! Thank you Smart & Final! The cost for 50 containers and 50 lids was less-than $20, so it works out to about $0.40 per container with lid, well worth it.

Before we start cutting our paper, let's laminate a set of color charts. I purchased a laminator, and although I don't use it that often, when I do use it, I am very glad that I have one. Lamination just adds life to your document or ID, or in this case, your color charts. Place the 0-13 color chart in the wallet-sized plastic sleeve and feed it through the laminator, repeat with the 6-8 color chart. Tape the two laminated color charts on the wall in your bathroom, somewhere near where you will be reading your pH. So when you wet the paper you hold it up to the chart, read it, then toss it. After a while you may find you don't really need to refer to the chart as you become familiar with the colors. But in the beginning, compare the paper to the color chart, because the better you monitor and record, the easier it will be to see patterns and draw conclusions.

Time to cut. Take a scissors and your 0-13 deli container and sit at a table with the open container in front of you. Pull about 6 feet of paper from the 0-13 roll and cut it. Now fold it in half to create 3 feet of 2-ply. Now fold it in half again, and you will have about 18 inches of 4-ply. Holding the paper near the end of one hand, and the scissors in the other, cut the paper in 1/4 inch strips, allowing the strips to fall into your deli container. It doesn't have to be exactly 1/4 inch. Just snip snip snip, then feed the paper forward, snip snip snip. Continue until you have cut the entire 18 inches of 4-ply. You should have approximately 288 strips of pH paper, 1/2 inch long by 1/4 inch wide. If you use 10 strips per day then this will last one month. If you use 5 strips a day, then two months. Now these strips may seem small, but when done correctly, you don't need a two-inch strip of paper. That's too wasteful. Done this way, your 288 strips cost about $1.50. So if it lasts you six weeks, then that's $1 a month. Repeat this cutting procedure for the 6-8 paper and deli container.

In the next chapter I will teach you how to use the paper and with practice you will be able to check your urine pH quickly with these ½ by ¼ inch strips, however, you are free to cut them any length you desire, just understand that the more you use the more you spend.

CHAPTER 12

TESTING

Now, this section gets a bit graphic, but we are all adults and it's not a big deal. But I want to help you do this and I've made all the errors so you don't have to.

There are two ways to test the pH of your urine. One way is to collect it in a container. In the beginning I used a 32oz deli container, the same as the previously-described deli container, just taller, like the two-pound cottage cheese containers, but clear plastic. This has the added benefit of allowing you to see color and clarity. My urine is always yellow or light yellow and clear. Anything that deviates from my normal color and clarity tells me that something may be wrong, especially if it persists or worsens. So since you can't see what's going on inside your body, you can at least get a clue by noticing what color and clarity your urine is. I don't routinely check this, but it's a good idea to know your normal urine color and clarity so you can recognize when it's not normal.

We discard urine down the bowl and never realize that this liquid just left our kidneys, which just came out of our blood, which just circulated throughout our entire body and organs. Urine color that is dark yellow or amber may be the result of foods you've eaten, or from lack of water (dehydration), or, from taking certain antibiotics or prescription medications that are "hard on the liver". The liver has to break down those medications, and according to the liver, it sees medications as toxic compounds. The first stage and first sign of liver damage is a change in urine color from yellow to amber that persists despite hydration and a changing diet.

So, the 32oz deli container is an ideal collection container in that it is wide enough for me to put my hand in partway and just touch the surface of the liquid with the paper. The liquid will run up the paper, so don't dip it, just make contact with the liquid and pull away. Remember, your paper is very small, ½ inch by ¼ inch. Hold the paper tightly at the edge with your index finger and thumb, and then just make contact with the liquid and pull away. The liquid will run up the paper about half or a quarter of the way and your fingers will remain dry. This will take some practice, that's true. Another thing you can do is, instead of touching the full 1/4-inch edge to the liquid, just touch the corner of the paper to the liquid. Again, don't dip. The liquid will travel up the paper. So, hold the paper tightly at the end, approach the liquid, as soon as you make contact with the corner, pull back. Don't Dip.

Hold the paper to the color chart, either on the wall or on the lid of the deli container, and compare.   Record your number. Congratulations!

Pour the urine from the container into the bowl, flush, rinse and towel dry the container and your hands, and you're done. See, not that hard.

You know, the hospitals have so much high-tech diagnostic equipment now, but it's interesting to note that the old-fashioned urine tests that haven't changed in decades have not gone away. In fact, done accurately, urine testing can tell you a lot of things, after all, this fluid just exited your kidneys and bloodstream.

When you get comfortable taking your pH from a container, try doing it midstream. Again, hold the paper tightly at one end, then just make contact with the stream, and pull back. Don't dip into the stream. As with the container technique, instead of touching the liquid with the full edge, just touch the stream with the corner of the paper. Remember that the liquid will travel up the paper.

With practice you will become a pro, and you can quickly check your urine pH without collecting it in a container, and eventually you'll know the colors and corresponding numbers so you won't use the color chart all the time either.

I did this diligently for about eight weeks, and then I drew my conclusions. I reprinted my weekly charts and highlighted 5s and 5.5s in pink, 6s with a yellow highlighter, and 7s with a green highlighter. I also recorded times of hard physical work. The patterns were easy to spot. The ABC Water kept me alkaline. When I finished my one quart, by evening my pH would fade south. In the morning, I'd wake up and it was 5. First thing I would do is drink 8 or 12 or even 16oz of ABC Water so that my next urination would be 6.8 or 7. Eventually, I decided to have 4-6oz of ABC Water one-hour before bed to ensure that my body had some alkalinity available to mop up the acid created during sleep.

I also noticed that when I did consume plenty of fruits and vegetables on any given day, that it did raise my pH. So it is true what they say, that an alkaline diet is a diet high in fruits and vegetables, no doubt about it, and that should be everyone's first choice for alkalinity.

But thank God for the bicarbonate in baking soda, for people like me who just don't get enough fruits and vegetables in their diet, and make matters worse with hard physical exercise and a few of life's mental stresses.

I cannot guide, advise, or help you beyond simply showing you how I personally did it. But I have provided you with ample material to refer to. In the beginning I couldn't believe how much baking soda I was consuming. I estimate that during the first three weeks I consumed about 2/3rds to 3/4ths of a cup of sodium-potassium bicarbonate. Now that was at a rate of 1.5 to 2 teaspoons a day, sipped on gradually throughout the day. But I was depleted in alkalinity, about a quarter tank remaining.

There's a book written about 100-years ago that describes the progressive signs of a body becoming more and more acidotic. I find it interesting that this was written so perceptively 100-years ago, and here we are today with not one person on television talking about this. And yet it's the foundation of health, the pH acid-alkaline status of your Internal Environment.

See if any of the following describes you or someone you know.
You think you are well, but you are not.
Do do do, go go go, you just can't stop.
Temperamental.
Unhappy about life and all you see.
Negative.
Can't get a good night's sleep.
Tired when you wake up and need caffeine to get you going.
Fatigue.
Symptoms of disease.

When I first read this, the first couple of descriptions made me think of the ADHD kids. How many vegetables and fruits are the ADHD kids eating? Conversely, how much acid-producing foods are they consuming, like colas, processed and junk foods, food colorings, preservatives, artificial sweeteners, toxic acid-forming hydrogenated or deep-fried fats. Then they are forced to sit when their bodies want to run, making their heads fill with anger and frustration. These poor kids. The adult world just doesn't understand what they're going through. You wouldn't expect a young growing child to be high in acid and low on alkaline, but I think we are witnessing this exact scenario in these kids.

Chapter Endnote
Throughout this book, chemical compounds are hyphenated, just be aware that the standard rule is to spell them as separate words. If you say them together, with the hyphen, the sentence should flow better. Hopefully!

CHAPTER 13

the Don'ts

Because bicarbonate is alkaline, you don't want to drink it 30 minutes before a meal or within 2 hours after a meal. Your stomach secretes hydrochloric acid in the presence of protein, and you don't want to disrupt this process. Now, this is not a hard-and-fast rule, as I have taken a few sips of ABC Water 10-15 minutes before a meal and not had any digestive issues. But to be safe, just go with the 30 minutes before and 2 hours after rule.

Should you experience gastrointestinal gurgling or worse, diarrhea, it is possible that you drank too much at one time. I can consume 16oz of ABC Water in less-than a minute and not experience any GI gurgling. Just don't drink too much too quickly. I would say no more than 8oz at once, this would be equal to 1/4t of sodium-potassium bicarbonate. If you buy baking soda from the household aisle instead of the baking aisle, well, that's your own fault. Household baking soda is not for consumption and not food grade. The impurities are likely what's making your stomach gurgle.

Like anything you eat or drink, your body should be in a calm relaxed state. Don't eat or drink anything, including ABC Water, if you are agitated, upset, excited, or while doing other tasks, i.e., multitasking.

The ABC Water is meant to be sipped gradually throughout the day, via the straw. Don't drink it from a glass like you would drink milk or juice.

Be sure to use clean sterile technique when making your ABC Water. While visiting someone, I once saw their cat walk across a section of the kitchen. Later, I saw that cat in the litter box.

Also, avoid leaving your water at room temperature. Water doesn't have any preservatives in it. Store your ABC gallons of water in the refrigerator, and when you're not drinking from your one-quart jar, put it in the refrigerator for later.

Don't continue drinking ABC Water if your urine pH is higher than 7. Whenever I see that my urine pH is 7.2, I just switch to plain water for the remainder of the day. If you see that your urine pH is 7.4, then skip ABC Water for a full day or more. ABC Water is only for when your urine pH is less-than 7. Remember, the target pH is exactly 7, not above, not below.

Don't be shy, tell people what you are drinking and refer them to this book. Don't give them the recipe. You can, but it's not fair to the author. If ABC Water™ has helped you, then support my book. It's the right thing to do. There was a time when I used to make a copy of a music CD if a coworker asked me to do so. What was I thinking? I wasn't thinking, obviously, autopilot. Not only is it illegal to do that, you short the artist of royalties for their work. Now I just casually tell them, "Just go online and buy a copy."

Don't do ABC Water if you have any kind of health problem. You need to be under the care of a doctor as health problems can become serious. This is not a medical book, it is a selfcare, do-it-yourself guide of my personal experience.

Don't go too fast at first. Recall that I started out with 75% of my urine pHs in the 5s, and so I started with a 1/2t of bicarb per day. One quart of ABC Water™ is 1t sodium-potassium bicarbonate, assuming your initial drinking-water is pH 5. If you want less, you can cut it in half by adding 16oz of ABC Water to your one-quart jar and top it with 16oz of plain water, and drink that gradually throughout the day. Your body has three pH buffering systems, like the gears in the transmission of your car. You want to take some time going from first gear to second gear, and then take some time to go from second gear to third gear. You can go quickly from first gear to third gear, just realize that the fast detoxification of your body might be unpleasant. For an ER patient presenting with severe acidosis, they don't waste any time getting that bicarb in. But any change of any kind should be done gradually.

Don't do your own thing. The ABC Water™ tastes fine, even good, because of the pure supplements and the recipe formulation. Plus, I've given you all the tools you need to determine your current acid alkaline status and my personal experience. As stated at the beginning of this book, JPM and the author are not liable for any harm or damages incurred by any and all readers. This is for informational purposes only and anything you do is by your own choice and you are personally responsible and liable for your own choices. This is another reason not to make copies of the recipe and hand them out to your friends. They need to read the book from cover to cover, and read it twice if necessary, to be sure they grasp all the aspects of acid-base balance and how ABC Water™ fits in.

CHAPTER 14

EXAMPLES

Below are five general categories that a person might see.

1. The Ammonia Urine Smell Person
This person is essentially 99% depleted in alkalinity, i.e., your car gasoline-empty light is red on the dashboard of your vehicle, indicating that, alert, alert, fill up now or your car could die in the middle of the street. Your urine pH may appear alkaline, 7 or above, but this is masking the true underlying acidosis. In order to survive and prevent your kidneys from being fried in acid, your body has taken to making ammonia, this is your emergency back-up system for neutralizing acid. If any of your urinations smell like ammonia, see your doctor. If this was me, I would slowly eliminate protein, exercise, and negative thinking, and I would slowly begin to eat cooked carrots and other cooked vegetables until the ammonia smell is gone. If that went well, I would juice fresh organic vegetables with every meal, along with lots of pure plain water. Basic Detox. Then I would slowly try the ABC Water in small amounts, gradually. The road to recovery should be taken gradually and slowly to allow the body time to adjust. Many people who don't eat well are walking around with one foot in the grave and don't recognize the seriousness of their condition. An ammonia urine, or breath, or body odor, is a medical red alert.

2. The Highly Acidic Person
Your initial urine-pH numbers at all times of the day were 5.

This person is alkaline depleted. It may take several weeks of drinking ABC Water to raise your urine pH up to 7 and able to keep it there. As in the ammonia case, go slowly to allow the body systems time to adjust and adapt. And remember, your diet is your best remedy. Fix it and feel better.

3. The Moderately Acidic Person
Your initial urine tests were, half 5s, half 6s, and the occasional 7.
This person is alkaline deficient. It may take two or more weeks of drinking ABC Water to get your urine pH up to 7 and able to keep it there. This person is likely struggling with their energy level. Seriously consider a vegan diet, or a partially-vegan diet, as you make your way to 7.

4. The Slightly Acidic Person
Your initial urine tests were, a few 5s, mostly 6s, and some 7s.
This person is low on alkaline reserves. It may take a few days to a week of drinking ABC Water to get your urine pH up to 7 and able to keep it there. This person is on the fence, not really in trouble, but could potentially go in that direction as time moves on. Review what you've been eating and look for ways to improve your diet to include more living plant food.

5. The Healthy Vegetarian
Your initial urine tests were, no 5s, half 6s and half 7s.
Good for you. If it was me, I would still aim to keep all my urine pHs at 7, and get those 6s up a bit. ABC Water can help fill in the gap where your fruits and vegetables aren't quite cutting it.

The Up Down Situation
If you notice that you are able to get your urine pH up to 7, but then your next urine pH is back down to 5 or 5.5, what's happening is that your body is sucking up all the alkalinity you are giving it. Your tissues are soaking it up like a sponge. I had this problem. I could drink 16oz of ABC Water in the morning and get my urine pH to jump up from 5 to 7, but then three hours later it would be right back down in the 5s again. My tissues were alkaline depleted, so any ABC Water that I consumed only made my urine

briefly alkaline, as the bulk of the bicarbonate was being soaked up by my acidic tissues, cells, and blood. But I was diligent and kept at it. Eventually, as stated before, at the end of the third week, my urine pH hit 7.4 and I realized that it was time to cut back from two quarts of ABC Water a day to one or one-and-a-half.

This is a completely individual experience, and I can't help you beyond showing you how to do it and telling you my own personal experience.

I will say though, that I think agencies are aware of the fact that many people are walking around in a partially-acidotic state, low or deficient in alkalinity. The reason I say this is because the fruits-and-vegetables recommendation seems to keep going higher and higher. First it was 3-5, then it was 5, then it was 5-7, and lately I've heard people say 7-9 servings of fruits and vegetables a day. So I think there are people out there that are aware that many people are alkaline deficient.

Another clue is the percent-fat and percent-carbohydrate recommendations. The percent-fat recommendation is 30%. That means that if you eat 2500 calories a day, then 30% of 2500 is 750. So you shouldn't be eating more than 750 calories of fat per day if you consume 2500 calories a day. For carbohydrates, I've seen labels that say 60% or your calories should be from carbohydrates. That means, no more than 1500 calories from carbohydrate if you eat 2500 calories a day. But they never say how much, or what your percent protein should be. However, since there are only three foods that have calories, fats, carbohydrates, and proteins, if fats are 30%, and carbs are 60%, then the protein is 10%. This, in my opinion, is a low protein diet, 10% of your total calories coming from protein. This is definitely a vegan-style diet, although vegans would be more like 70% carbs, 15% fat, and 15% protein.

So, the news and the media are trying to get us to eat 7-9 servings of fruits and vegetables, up from 3-5, and cut back our protein to 10%. This is an alkaline diet approach. Could it be that some agency believes we have an alkaline deficiency epidemic going on?

I would say so.

Having spent the past 20+ years performing lab tests for hospitals, I estimate that 80% of all the urines I tested had a pH of 5 or 5.5, and the other 19% being 6 or 6.5, and about 1% of the people had a 7 urine pH. Again, just because something is COMMON it doesn't mean it's NORMAL. I worked seven years at a cardiac hospital and 99% of the urines had a pH of 5. And it wasn't the machine because I checked the test strips visually to make sure. All of these things and experiences have brought me to write this book, in hopes that this "step-by-step solution to Alkaline Deficiency™" will help people who, like me, simply have more acid production going on than alkaline coming in.

Oh, there is one other group besides healthy vegetarians that have a urine pH of 7. It's the healthy newborn babies. Who enter the world perfectly created.

Chapter Endnote
I would like to emphasize that nearly all the urines from patients at the cardiac hospital had a pH of 5. The medical system will never piece this together and reveal it. Keep in mind that when you enter a hospital for treatment, you see the nurse, you see the doctor, you see a phlebotomist, and perhaps a radiologist or respiratory therapist. But you rarely see the Clinical Laboratory Scientist, the person in the lab, the person not only familiar with your lab test numbers, but the person who is actually generating those numbers.

CHAPTER 15

the Vegan

The vegan diet should be the first choice for providing your body with alkalinity. Seventh-Day Adventists who follow the vegetarian recommendations of Ellen White are known to live longer and healthier lives that those who don't. The problem is, for most of us, there are just too many other tempting, delicious, nonplant foods that we are not willing to part from. Having contemplated this, I am a believer of the positive health claims of an all-plant diet, however, I don't believe human beings are exclusive plant eaters, but rather, that human beings are omnivores, eating both plant and animal foods, and this, of course, is also taught in schools.

Most vegans are aware that they have to supplement with vitamin B12 because a vegan diet does not provide sufficient B12, which is found in meat, fish, poultry, eggs, and dairy. So if our Creator wanted us to be 100% vegetarian, where would we get sufficient vitamin B12 from?

Additionally, a vegan diet consists of a lot of starches, corn, rice, pasta, potatoes. Starches, also called staples, are basically just inexpensive highly-concentrated fuel. A steady diet of starches creates a soft-muscle-tissue type of body. The muscles are soft because they are mixed with fat. If we could wave a magic wand, most of us would choose to have hard lean muscles, and this is more likely achieved by including a combination of animal and plant foods in your diet.

Some people who are ill or have a health crisis turn to a 100% plant diet in an attempt to heal themselves. Many people report success in doing so. The primary reason, I believe, is due to stopping the consumption of acid-producing foods, and eating a diet exclusively of alkaline-producing foods. They fix their acid-base balance. They tip the scales back in the other direction, where they should be. The alkaline foods mop up the acid in their body raising their pH. The problem I see is that most people don't do it long enough. If your body is failing, your blood, tissues, intracellular fluids, are on empty with regard to alkalinity. A week of juicing isn't going to stock you up. You'll feel better, but you'll only be running on an eighth of a tank. Juice daily and eat a vegan diet for a year or more and you'll be more likely to fix your acidosis. But, if that's not possible, the next best option is to supplement with bicarbonate for a source of alkalinity.

There is a third option, and that is, the mixed approach. Eat more fruits and vegetables and supplement with bicarbonate every other day. This is an entirely individual decision that only the reader can design for themselves. After they've determined their current acid alkaline status. Using pH paper. Testing and recording all of his or her urinations.

Another problem I personally have with the vegan diet is that high starch component again. Starches are just long chains of sugars, glucose molecules. I used to make mashed potatoes with mushroom gravy as a meal, no meat, no fat. It was 350 calories. Then I noticed I would get the shakes five minutes after eating it. Well no duh. This meal is an extremely high glycemic load, 300 calories of starch, 40 calories of protein, and 10 calories of fat. Those 300 calories of finely mashed potato starch were quickly converted into 300 calories of glucose sugar. What was I thinking? Well, I was doing the best with the knowledge I had at the time. I've learned a lot since then. The vegan diet is essentially a diet whereby you carb-load every single day of your life. It's just too high in carbs and low in protein for me.

Now, it doesn't hurt to give yourself one day during the week when you eat mostly fruits and vegetables. I do this. I call it, NCD Fat Free Sunday™. I eat bananas and oranges, grapes and whatever fruits are in season at the time. But I don't eat any fat on this day, because the high sugar means high insulin, and as already stated, insulin takes excess sugar and converts it into body fat. But to make things worse, if dietary fat is present, insulin takes the sugar and converts it to body fat, and then takes the dietary fat and converts it to body fat. A double whammy! This is why desserts, such as ice cream, cheesecake, whole-milk pudding, carrot cake, all of which are about half fat calories and half sugar calories, are so dangerous to your waistline. The sugar raises insulin and the whole thing gets converted into body fat.

But the low-protein high-plant diet does create an alkaline environment within the body, and this is a good thing. Additionally, all the phytonutrient color pigments, detoxifying plant fiber, and living enzymes and natural minerals, makes this diet an ideal choice for nutritional support, cleansing, and body repair.

Chapter Endnote
The words Vegan and Vegetarian are sort of loosely used when you talk to people. Vegans don't eat any animal products or wear leather or fur, they are the PETA people, people for the ethical treatment of animals. Vegetarians may eat dairy or eggs. Most people who call themselves "vegetarians" don't eat dairy or eggs, or very rarely, but because they wear leather shoes or belts, they can't call themselves vegans. I use the words interchangeably, but just be aware of the difference.

Vegans don't eat or wear animals, aka, the "strict vegetarian".
Vegetarians don't eat animals but own clothing made from them.
Lacto-Vegetarian – a vegetarian that eats dairy.
Ovo-Vegetarian – a vegetarian that eats eggs.
Lacto-Ovo-Vegetarian – a vegetarian that eats dairy and eggs.
Lacto-Ovo-Meat-Vegetarian – the NCD! You get to eat (and wear) whatever you want!

CHAPTER 16

Vitamin B&C

There are great benefits to taking vitamin B and C gradually throughout the day. Vitamin B is like your energy vitamin, being required for many reactions in the body that produce energy. It's also the anti-stress vitamin. If you need a pick-me-up, instead of turning to caffeine, try a little vitamin B, and the ABC Water™ is the ideal way to do this.

One quart of ABC Water has 1/4th capsule of B100 complex. This doesn't sound like much, but it's enough. You don't want to use any more than one capsule per gallon of water, per the ABC Water™ recipe, because vitamin B doesn't taste good in large amounts.

Vitamin C is the wonder vitamin, in that, it is your tissue healer and your body's primary water-soluble antioxidant. So, as damage is being done to your body hour by hour, from pollution, the metabolism of food, and just everyday activities, your body's vitamin C is busy fixing everything and trying to revert tissues and cells back to new again.

So as you can see, this formulation is, in my opinion, perfect. I wouldn't add anything to it, although you could, but things like minerals, magnesium, calcium, etc., are best added to your food, rather than to your water, to ensure you are getting your minerals. Adding minerals to the ABC Water makes it too thick and gritty, even with very finely-ground mineral supplements. If you are thinking of adding herbs to the ABC Water, well, you could, but they are better taken with food or alone, or according to the manufacturer's recommendations.

The ABC Water™ is perfect as is. The only thing you might want to do is increase or decrease the amount of sodium-potassium bicarbonate, depending on what your alkaline needs are. To decrease the bicarbonate by half, just cut the number of teaspoons in half, or you could pour 16oz of ABC Water into your 32oz drinking jar and top it off with 16oz of plain water. To increase the amount of bicarbonate supplementation, rather than add more bicarbonate to the ABC Water recipe, just increase the amount of ABC Water you drink to one-and-a-half quarts, but this is entirely a personal choice depending on your own personal acid alkaline status, as determined by your current and historical urine-pH numbers. If you do decide to tweak the amount of sodium-potassium bicarbonate in the ABC Water to meet your individual needs, just be sure to always check your urine pH throughout the day, aiming to keep it at exactly 7, not higher, not lower. Higher is going to give you that headache faint feeling because you're getting too much, and lower is going to move you in the direction of fatigue, so 7 exactly, pH neutral, the pH of plain water.

Now you might be thinking, I'm not going to purchase vitamin B and C from drclarkstore.com, I'm just going to use what I have, or some other brand. Well, you may not like the taste of the brand you have. Plus, it may not dissolve entirely. Then there's the question of how much of another brand to use. And impurities, that's the most important reason of all. If you are going to drink this every day you are going to want to know that your vitamins B and C are the purest available.

I once brought my NCD Hawaiian Pizza™ to a potluck, and it was a huge hit. When asked what's in it, I said "it's a secret", as I knew then that one day I would be publishing my recipes. Later, one of the ladies told me she tried to make it at home but it didn't taste the same. That's because "you didn't have the recipe" I said.

CHAPTER 17

THE RECIPE

Let's assume you have all of your ingredients, your glass gallon bottles, and your one-quart drinking jar with straw. Time to make some ABC Water!

Line your four, one-gallon glass bottles in a row on the counter and place a six-inch wide funnel in the top of the first bottle.

Using your measuring spoons, add 2.5t of sodium bicarbonate to the bottle, that's one level teaspoon twice, and then a level half-teaspoon. Repeat with the second, third, and fourth bottles, moving the funnel as you go. Put the baking soda away.

Repeat with the potassium bicarbonate, 2.5t per bottle, one two three four bottles, then put the $KHCO_3$ away.

Add one cap of B100 to each bottle, pulling the capsule apart by holding it at the ends and then rolling the capsule back-and-forth to expel the powder. Toss the empty gel caps in the trash, and put away the vitamin B.

Add a level 1/2 measuring teaspoon of vitamin C powder to each gallon, or two caps if you bought the capsules. Put the vitamin C away.

Now add your water. Fill it to about two inches from the top. If it fizzes a little, stop and move on to the next bottle, you can come back to it in a minute. When you have all of your bottles filled, blot the mouth of the bottles with a clean towel and screw on the caps, hand tighten. Invert each bottle 6x to mix, then place them in your refrigerator. Allow them to completely dissolve overnight before drinking.

2.5t sodium bicarb
2.5t potassium bicarb
1cap B100
1/2t vitamin C
Add water, wipe, cap, mix, refrigerate.

Dividing one gallon into 4 gives you:
1t sodium-potassium bicarbonate (assuming your water is pH 5)
1/4cap vitamin B complex
570mg vitamin C

Here's a bonus, the ascorbic acid will become ascorbate in the presence of bicarbonate. This is a more absorbable form of vitamin C and is easier on the digestive tract than ascorbic acid. One reference I read said that vitamin C in its base form, (ascorbate), goes directly to the adrenal glands for adrenal support. If this is true, this would make ascorbate a cortisol crusher! Cortisol being a catabolic hormone, and the opposite of what all athletes want, which is anabolism.

So, in addition to the B complex vitamins providing stress relief, the vitamin C in its ascorbate form is also providing stress relief through adrenal gland support. THAT'S AMAZING!!

"ANABOLIC" ASCORBATE, THE CORTISOL CRUSHER™

This is another reason why the ABC Water™ recipe formulation is so fantastic, and why I've made it the Number One thing, top-of-the-list, what people should be doing.

Below is an example of how your day might look.

06:00 up, 8 sips 8oz of ABC Water
07:00 Breakfast
08:00
09:00
10:00 8 sips of ABC Water
11:00 Lunch
Noon
13:00
14:00 4 sips of ABC Water
15:00 Snack or Meal Shake
16:00
17:00 8 sips ABC Water
18:00 Dinner
19:00
20:00
21:00 4 sips, the remainder of the 32oz ABC Water
22:00 lights out

Try to save 4 to 6 or even 8 ounces of ABC Water for one-hour before bed. This will give your body the vitamin B and C and alkalinity it needs to do its nightly cleanup and repair. If you can get that first morning urine to be in the high 6s or ideally, exactly 7, then, if your experience is like mine, you'll have zero morning fatigue.

Another secret to reducing morning fatigue, and that need for a cup of caffeine to get you going, is to have a little protein before bed. No carbs, just two ounces of chicken breast, which is about 75 calories. Cooked chicken weighs about 15-25% less-than raw chicken, depending on the cooking method. Therefore, 2oz cooked is about 2.5oz raw, and 4oz of raw chicken breast is 120 calories.

So, have 6oz of ABC Water one-hour before bed. Then, 30 minutes after the ABC Water, have the chicken. Now your bloodstream is charged with amino acids, vitamin B, vitamin C, and alkalinity, and it can go to work cleaning and repairing so that when morning comes, you hit the ground running! You heard it here first.

CHAPTER 18

Shortcut

I never take shortcuts on something that's important. So if you've read this far you may be thinking, "No kidding he didn't take any shortcuts, this is way too involved for my busy schedule." Well, for those of you that want to do this but don't have the time, here are some suggestions.

If you eat protein with every meal, bacon and eggs for breakfast, double cheeseburger for lunch, three-piece chicken meal for dinner, and you consume 0-3 servings of fruits and vegetables a day, you might try adding a 1/2t of baking soda to some water and drink it every day, or Monday Wednesday Friday, and see how it makes you feel. If this was me, that's what I would do. You could also buy one roll of pH paper from amazon.com for about $12 and start testing your urine pH to see if it's almost always 5, or half the time 5, or sometimes 5, or occasionally 5. Perhaps once you begin to see that your urine pH is never 7, that you will invest some time on the weekend to set up the ABC Water™ as described here, and take your acid alkaline status seriously. No doctor can do this for you. Their expertise is to identify your disease then write out a prescription for it. If you have a good doctor, he might privately tell you that, yeah, a lot of people's underlying problem is simple acidosis.

If you do eat three servings of vegetables a day and your protein consumption is as described above, if I was this person and was short on time, I would probably start taking 1/4t baking soda every day. But I would still buy some pH paper online and see what the alkaline status is of that liquid exiting my kidneys. If you are acidotic, I doubt that you would even notice any improvement with 1/4t, maybe. I have no idea what your condition is and I cannot advise you in any way, shape or form, other than to say that if it was me I would spend $12 and a little bit of time getting to know my body's alkaline status. It's no different than taking control of your weight or your finances.

If I had to put a number on it, I would say, for me personally, that 1/8th of a measuring teaspoon of baking soda probably has the alkalinity equal to 125 calories of fresh fruit, so like, two small oranges, or one medium pear or banana, seven ounces of grapes, 15oz of watermelon. But, that's based solely on my personal experience from observing how my diet affects my urine pH.

Again, I am not telling you to do anything. You, as an adult, are free to decide what to do with this information. This chapter was merely to give an example of what I would personally do if I was in said situation, or if a family member said to me, "What's the quickie way?" For me, there is no shortcut method. But I also understand that there are people who would like to do this but don't have a lot of free time in their schedule and that it's human nature to think of a shortcut and then someone devises a shortcut plan that could be potentially harmful, and so this chapter provides a reasonable shortcut example of what I would do if it was me.

For the sodium-potassium bicarbonate, I have a shortcut for this as well. Go to www.drclarkstore.com again, and type "balanced bicarb" in the search-box. You will see a half-cup bag of sodium-potassium bicarb for $8.79. One bag will supply enough to make about 3.5 gallons of ABC Water, that's 14 quarts, or in my case, about a two-week supply. I was buying this but it was costing almost $20 a month. However, when I look at all the things people spend money on, $2500 for a 4-day cruise, for example, would cost the same as ten years of this balanced-bicarb product. So the question becomes, do you want four days of fun, or ten years of alkalizing your body for optimum health? For me the answer is an easy one, and I may start buying this product and phasing out the Trader Joe's sodium bicarbonate and Nuts.com potassium bicarbonate, or I may alternate, one batch of ABC Water using DrClarkStore's balanced bicarb, and the next batch using Trader Joe's and Nuts.com.

In any case, for those of you who want a sodium-potassium bicarb, this Balanced Bicarb product can be added to your drclarkstore order, then you don't have to bother with supermarket baking soda or ordering from nuts.com.

Chapter Endnote
While researching grammar and spelling, I came across this example with regard to hyphen use. Try to avoid the stringing-together-of-lots-of-words-and-ideas tendency.

Also, in case you aren't current with informal spellings, I wasn't, here are a few you might find helpful.
ya = you
yeah = yes
yah = a British word for an upper-class person
yay! = hooray! great!
yea = yes, opposite of nay

CHAPTER 19

STRATEGY

So, for those of you that want to do this, let me help you come up with a strategy, strategery.

You work a job, you earn vacation time. If you take a week off, use three days to go on vacation with your family, then take a couple of days to "do a project".

The day before you leave for vacation, go online and place your orders for B100, vitamin C powder, potassium bicarbonate, a case of glass one-gallon bottles and caps, and if you want to drink out of a one-quart glass jar, order a case with the lids. You can use a plastic straw, but why not go for the glass straw and be the talk of the neighborhood.

Then go to your healthfood store or grocery store and buy your baking soda from the baking aisle. Transfer it to a bigger jar to make it user-friendly as the original container's opening is likely to be too small. I use a wide-mouth 16-ounce glass jar with screw cap, the same type as the 32-ounce jar. Use a label maker to print a label and label it $NaHCO_3$ or Baking Soda. A label maker is a "must-have" if you like to keep things organized and neat. The shelves, trays, and containers in my refrigerator are all labeled. I use the Dymo Letra Tag available at Walmart for $16, along with the 2-pack paper tape for $8. Don't buy the fancy label makers that cost $60 as the tapes are way expensive.

Next, buy your pH paper, either the five rolls of the two types, or if you want to search amazon.com or Ebay for single rolls that's up to you. Just remember, that the jumbo rolls are a half inch wide, so you can cut them in ¼ inch increments, resulting in small ½ x ¼ inch strips. This is the most economical.

Obtain two deli containers for the two types of pH-paper strips. Either buy two small eight-ounce plastic deli containers from a deli, or a big roll from a restaurant-supply store like Smart & Final, or find something from around your house, but get them ready so that you can set up your containers when your pH paper arrives, keeping your momentum going.

Create a weekly tracker form. You can do this on a computer or the old-fashioned way by just drawing a grid with a ruler. Use cardstock so that it's easier to record and read your numbers as plain-weight paper tends to curl up on the ends. Buy a clipboard, and three pens, red, blue, green.

Okay, you're done. Go enjoy your 3-day vacation!

One Two Three Four, you're back, and your orders have arrived. Break the seals on your B100 and vitamin C powder, write the date on them and put them in your refrigerator. The vitamin C says "store in a dark dry place, do not refrigerate" but I refrigerate all my supplements. The cool temperature keeps the nutrients from degrading, and I don't put hot food in a cold refrigerator, creating humidity. But that's what I do, it's your choice.

Transfer your potassium bicarbonate to a 16-ounce glass jar and label it $KHCO_3$, or Potassium Bicarbonate. The entire contents of the one-pound bag from nuts.com will fill the 16oz jar, with a little left over that you will use for your first batch of ABC Water.

Now let's do the pH paper. Remove the rolls from their containers, don't remove the foil from the rolls. Each roll comes with a color chart so you will have five of each, set them aside. Using your vacuum sealer, seal four rolls of each type of paper, one roll per bag. You don't want your pH paper to be exposed to humidity. Label and date them and place them in a brown-paper bag for additional protection from light. Now take the 6-8 roll, remove it from the foil and pull six feet, cut it, fold it in half, fold it in half again. Begin cutting ¼ inch strips into the deli container. When you're done, tape the 6-8 color chart to the inside of the deli lid. Repeat with the 0-13 paper. You're doing Awesome!!!!!

Okay, you're all set. Take a break and then we'll make the ABC Water.

Your one-gallon bottles have arrived, so take them out of the box and rinse them and the caps, and towel dry. Aren't they nice? I think so. Line them up on the counter and place a funnel in the first one. I make 4 gallons at a time, 16 quarts, a two-week supply.

Check the pH of your drinking-water and adjust the following teaspoon amounts accordingly (see Chapter 3).

Add 2.5 level measuring teaspoons sodium bicarbonate to each bottle. Put it back in the fridge.
Add 2.5 level measuring teaspoons potassium bicarbonate to each bottle. Put it back in the fridge.
Add ½ a level measuring teaspoon of the vitamin C powder to each bottle. Put it back in the fridge.
Take four capsules of B100. While holding the capsule over the funnel, pull the capsule apart and roll the gel cap between your fingers to expel the orange powder. Toss the empty gel cap, and repeat with the remaining bottles.

Now fill the bottles with water, either your reverse-osmosis water from your tap, or your reverse-osmosis water that you bought at the supermarket, or your spring water from your five-gallon hard-plastic water bottle that you purchased from a bottling company. Leave an inch or two of air at the top. If there is fizzing, wait one minute and then continue. Cap each bottle tightly, invert six times to mix, then refrigerate. Allow it to dissolve completely by letting it sit overnight.

Last step. Wash and dry three of your new one-quart jars and lids. Grab the drill and insert a 3/8ths drill bit. With the cap right-side up, place the tip in the center and gently drill a hole. Smooth out the hole with a cloth, and repeat with two more lids. Clean up. Wash and dry your glass straw, flicking out the water from the inside and standing it up somewhere in a corner to allow the interior to air-dry.

Now, the water isn't going to spoil in the refrigerator, so spend the next seven days testing and recording ALL of your urinations so that you can determine your current alkaline status before you begin drinking your ABC Water. Remember, your goal is to simply use the ABC Water to bump your urine pH up to 7. If it's already at 7, then you don't need any additional alkalinity. Review or reread this book from the beginning if you're not fully sure.

Chapter Endnote
The verb "to air dry" is transitioning to "air-dry". Dictionaries have the verb form hyphenated, but it hasn't fully caught on.

CHAPTER 20

TRACKING

Wouldn't it be nice if we could track our vitamin C levels or our vitamin D levels or our tissue magnesium level, in order to see if our bodies are low or not? Fortunately, you do have a way to test and track your body's acid alkaline status.

In order to see patterns and to make correlations between how you feel and your urine pH, you will need to test and record all of your urinations for several weeks or months until you come to know yourself. Make several copies of your weekly chart and clip them to your clipboard. Test and record throughout the day, every day, and then review at the end of the week. Make notations or keep a journal, include things like, exercise, times when you worried, high-protein dinners, high fruit-and-vegetable days. The more you put into it, the more likely it is that you will begin to see patterns and relationships between how you feel and your urine pH. This is called Tracking. If you just make a mental note and try to store it all in your head, by the end of the week you won't have seen any patterns or made much correlation. Believe me, when you have 35 numbers on a weekly grid, and eight weeks of data, the patterns jump out at you. So don't track in your head. Use the red blue green pens and your charts.

Below are the patterns I discovered for myself.

1. I would go to bed with a urine pH of 7 and wake up with a 5.

Solution, ABC Water one-hour before bed.

2. The bottoms of my feet would be achy when I got out of bed if my morning pH was 5, slightly-achy feet if I woke up with a 6, and a bounce in my step with no achy soles of feet if I woke up with a urine pH of 7. Achy joints, hands, feet, muscles, back, that's often excess acid that hasn't been mopped up.

3.   After 30-45 minutes of weightlifting, my urine pH would PLUNGE. That's when I added my first amendment to my daily one quart, that for every 30 minutes of hard physical work or 60 minutes of moderate physical work, I drink an additional 16oz of ABC Water. One textbook states that lactic acid levels in the muscles can increase to twelve-times normal immediately after hard exercise. This is why exercising when your body's already acidic is dangerous. The acid on top of acid could potentially tip you over the edge, as what occurred to James Fixx, the man credited for making jogging popular with his book, *The Complete Book of Running*. He died of a heart attack at the age of 52 after his daily run, and apparently he had a stressful job and had gone through two divorces. If only he, and so many others, had known about acid and the criticalness of acid-alkaline balance. If you already have acid or fatigue, i.e., you are not fully recovered from your previous workout, and you work out again, you add acid on top of acid.   When what you should be doing is recovering; hydration,   nutrition,   sleep,   light-movement   exercise,   and alkalization.   Acid on top of acid, will just put your body in a Catabolic Cortisol state. The exact opposite of what you want. Steroid-using athletes don't take catabolic hormones, they take anabolic hormones, growth hormones. And here's what people commonly do, they mask their acidic state with caffeine, and zoom zoom zoom, off we go to the gym to work out. That's cheating, and you will know it when two hours after the workout you are in a complete CRASHED state. Your body wasn't ready to work out again. It hadn't regained its alkaline state of freshness.

4. I also noticed that if I skipped a day or two of ABC Water, that I had to take extra the next couple of days to catch up. This is when

I added the adjective RELIGIOUSLY to my rule. One quart of ABC Water daily, Religiously. Because if I skip days, my urine pH starts to drop back down to 5 again, and I don't like 5.

5. I saw a bit of an "alkaline tide" at 10:00 but it was random. Science hasn't confirmed the phenomenon, other than to say that it can occur after a meal or at certain times of the day. Tide or no tide, I just aim at keeping my urine pH as close to 7 as possible. Think of a dart board, you want to keep landing your dart in the center of the bull's eye, 7.

6. And then I recently discovered that if I fail to brush off an offense, and I inadvertently take that offense with me when I go to sleep, I will wake up with a urine pH of 5. And it may take me half the day to get my pH back up to 7 and able to keep it there. Offenses come, it's just a part of life, to test what you're made of, and how you respond. Brush them off. Actually, that's not exactly right. Picture someone throwing a dart at you, and you feel it hit you in the rear shoulder, ouch! Don't just "brush it off" exactly. But rather, pull the dart out, then LOOK at the person who threw it, then open your hand, drop the dart on the floor, and walk away. I used to just brush off offenses by certain offenders, but then they would turn around the next week and do it again. That's when, I began to LOOK at them, SEE them, and then brush it off. That sends a different message to the offender. The last thing you want to do is absorb an offense. When you absorb an offense it now lives in you and it can activate your physiology without you even being aware of it. Acid is being produced and you can't figure out the source. Your blood pressure is up and you don't know why. Here's why. You let something, or someone, get to you. See Ephesians 6.11 if this is you.

Those were my correlations.
My conclusions are as follows.

1. Acidosis causes me to feel fatigued.

2. Alkalosis and a urine pH of 7 gives me almost endless energy.

3. Raising the pH of my urine to 7 lowered my blood pressure.

4. One foot in the grave begins with the depletion of my alkaline reserves.

Chapter Endnote
Grammarians say, if the first word of the compound adjective ends in "-ly" then no hyphen is needed. But there are exceptions to this rule. Some of you may not have noticed, but you'll see it happen again later on. You'll be an expert in grammar by the end of this!

CHAPTER 21

High Protein

We looked at the high-alkaline diet of the vegetarian, now let's look at the high-protein diet, commonly referred to as the Atkins Diet. The principle is sound, that is, cut carbs, and especially sugar carbs, and the fat falls off. The problem is that at a certain point, you become so carb depleted that all of a sudden, one day, you blow it and start eating carbs. Then the next day, you continue eating carbs, and more carbs, and pretty soon you've eaten all the carbs that you've been depriving yourself of over the past six weeks. Hence, the term, "Yo-Yo Dieting", where you lose weight only to gain it all back again, plus some extra.

The second problem behind this protein and fat diet, or ProFat diet, is that the food choices were very heart risky. By that I mean, people were eating steak with beef fat, whole chicken with chicken fat, pork ribs and bacon with pork fat, half a dozen eggs with egg-yolk fat, cheese, butter, sour cream, and more protein. It's the "Heart-Attack" diet. You've heard of the Heart-Attack Grill restaurant in Las Vegas, where a man died of a heart attack while eating the Triple-Bypass Burger. It's funny but it's not. The burger is 6000 calories of animal fat and protein, enough calories for three days, eaten at one sitting. Crazy.

We all enjoy a nice juicy burger or steak, but you have to balance out your meal with some carbs and especially some alkalizing vegetables so that your body can cope with all the acid-producing protein.   And definitely control your calories per meal, 6000 is insane. I rarely eat more than 1000 calories at one sitting and 95% of the time my meals are 500 calories. The JPM recipes, Number Crunched Meals™, are designed so that each of the recipes divides into a certain number of meals, and each meal is 500 calories. This makes CALORIE COUNTING MADE EASY™ because you don't count calories, you count PRE-COUNTED MEALS™.

So if I have five meals a day, I had 2500 calories. If I have six meals, I had 3000 calories. If I had four meals and a half meal, I had 2250 calories.

Fat Loss Is A Numbers Game.™ When you take control of the numbers, you take control of your weight.

It's other things as well, macronutrients (percent macros), sugar load (glycemic load), fiber, food additives, artificial chemicals, yeast infections, worm infections, normal gut flora, thyroid function, mineral status, vitamin status, how fast you eat, how much you chew, and on and on. But primarily, it's all numbers.

I find it interesting that so many of the "experts" say not to count calories, it's too difficult and takes too much time and you don't need to if you just do this certain trick. Trick is right. They are tricking millions of people out of their money every year.

I came up with my own plan for weight maintenance and fat loss because I wanted something that gave me lots of control, lots of freedom, and that worked. The NCD™ is that plan, and I've been revising it for over a decade, so that the finished product is ready for publication. I think you will find it's a New and Unique approach that makes a lot of sense.

To summarize then, the macros for the vegan diet are 70% carbs, 15% fat, and 15% protein, and at the other end of the spectrum, the ProFat diet is 20% carbs, 40% fat, and 40% protein, and in the initial Induction Phase, it's 10% carbs and 90% profats. I am not a big fan of extremes. But, if you are ill, you need an alkaline vegan diet, and if you are obese then you need a low-carb ProFat diet. Extreme situations do require extreme measures. But for the rest of us who are somewhere in the middle, how about a diet plan that is moderate carbs, moderate fat, and moderate protein. This approach is really the diabetic diet. And technically, we should all be taking the diabetic approach to eating, that is, moderate carbs, not high carbs, not low carbs, and moderate fat, not high fat, not low fat, and moderate protein, not high protein, not low protein.

Since we need fats for cell membranes and steroid hormones, and we need protein for enzymatic reactions, cell structure, and muscle, and we need glucose for cellular energy and brain function, doesn't it make sense that we should be getting a balance of all three at each meal? I think so. It makes sense to me. The macros then, that I target my meals to be, are 40% carbs 30% fat and 30% protein, almost a third a third a third, with a slight tip towards the carbs.

Now you can tweak this to achieve certain objectives, such as, to lose a little fat, drop your carbs to 30% and raise your fats to 40%, so 30% carbs 40% fat 30% protein. Some bodybuilding books have 40% protein meals, which just becomes too much protein after a while. You can eat a 40% protein meal once or maybe twice a day, but not five times a day every day.

If you want to add a little size to your muscles, drop the fat to 20% and increase your carbs to 50%, so 50% carbs 20% fat 30% protein. See how I said "tweak" as opposed to "radically shift". Your body won't notice small tweaks, but it will notice radical shifts. And when you radically shift to something, the natural homeostatic response is for your body to radically shift back to where it was. Hence the yo-yo dieting phenomenon that so many people, including myself, have experienced. This same principle of homeostasis, applies to getting healthy when you are sick. If you radically shift to a healthy way of life and diet, your body will want to radically shift back to its diseased state. This is why you have to make changes gradually, so that you sort of fool your body into this or that. An example of this is, suppose you weigh 130 lbs, and then you gain 10 lbs to 140 lbs. At the beginning, you can fairly easily drop the extra 10 lbs and get back to 130 lbs again, because your body still thinks it's 130 lbs. However, as time goes on, and you stay at 140 lbs, now your body says, "okay, I'm 140 lbs now" and so losing that extra 10 lbs is harder because you waited and your body's homeostasis or "current state" shifted. We see this with chronic disease also. Someone appears to be fine, and then is diagnosed with XYZ disease, and they never come out of it. They will stay with XYZ disease until the end. The disease condition didn't happen overnight, the official diagnosis happened overnight, but the condition occurred gradually. Your body moved gradually into a diseased state, so too must it move gradually back to a healthy state, if the healthy state is to become permanent. So it is with PERMANENT fat loss. Radical change is much harder to hold on to for the long term.

You have to fool or trick your body so that it doesn't notice. That's why the NCD approach works. It's moderate moderate moderate, and then to achieve a bit more of a desired result, you tweak the macro percentages a bit.

How this fits with acidosis and alkalosis is, the 30%-protein meals are a moderate protein, moderate acid-producing diet. The Atkins, or ProFat diet, is a high acid-producing diet, and without sufficient fruits and vegetables, you run the risk of having a coronary event should you decide to stay on it long term, (several weeks to several months). However, there is a way of getting around this high-protein high-acid diet, and that is, to supplement with alkalinity via the ABC Water, in lieu of sufficient dietary fruits and vegetables.

CHAPTER 22

Chicken or the Egg

We looked at the "What Came First, the Chicken or the Egg" earlier in this book, but let's look at it again so that we grasp the importance of how our internal environment plays a key role in our health or lack thereof.

Now the man who died of a heart attack eating the burger, did his heart just give way and explode? Or did the burger tip the scales of his internal environment, and this tipping of the scales of his internal environment cause his heart to explode? The autopsy will say, coronary arrest. But what about the underlying symptoms? My theory is, that this person was already running on empty with regard to alkalinity. I wouldn't have been surprised if his urinations had the smell of ammonia for the past few months. He is walking around in an acidic state. He sits down, starts eating a large amount of animal protein, and animal fat, what would be referred to as a "heavy" meal, and before long, the production of acid tips the scales beyond their capacity, and boom, complete body shutdown. I wouldn't be surprised if the autopsy report also stated, kidney, liver, pancreas, gall bladder, spleen, and lung failure as well as heart failure.

Let's look at why two people in a household come down with the flu while two other people in the same household do not. All of them are being exposed to the same germs, viruses, bacteria, the same doorknobs, the same air, the same towels, etc. Why didn't the other two people get sick? Well, your answer might be, "The other two were healthier, and the two that got sick were run-down, or already compromised." Well, what does healthy mean? What does compromised mean exactly? What constitutes a healthy state? What constitutes a compromised state? Your immune system, yes, that's part of it. If you have a chronic health problem, then your immune system is always on and over time it gets run-down. But go back a step further and ask, "What caused your chronic health problem?"

There are many things that contribute to a health problem and it's never as simple as just one thing. But I will say this, initial health problems begin, or take hold, or take root, because the internal environment is not primed with alkalinity, but rather tipping towards acidosis. I believe, this compromise in acid-base balance is the starting point for all the other compromises that will follow.

Let me say that again. I believe, the compromise in acid-base balance in the body is the starting point for all other compromises that will follow.™

The autopsy report of the coronary arrest is the surface, outward presentation of the problem, heart failure, organ failure, the "Chicken" you might say. I say the real problem was below the surface, at the level of the fluids, that precious fluid that bathes the organs, the "Egg" if you will. It's the same as your car. The mechanic says, "The transmission's dead." Then you ask, "How did that happen?" He replies, "Your fluid's burnt." Then you say, "Oh, so I have to keep the fluid pink or my transmission will burn out."

It's a hard lesson to learn, but you take the financial blow to your wallet and continue on, a bit more informed. For the heart-attack person who died while eating the 6000-calorie triple-bypass burger, he never got a chance to learn, he's just done.

Here's something else I noticed about medical care. They will say, they don't know how this or that happens, but they know your diet has nothing to do with it. Well, if you don't know the cause, how do you know that diet is not the cause? Well, now they are starting to say that diet is the cause because the public is not fooled by that line anymore, that, "We don't know the cause but it's not related to your diet." Just keep eating, drinking, and doing all of those things that aren't good for you, it has nothing at all to do with this particular disease. Good grief. I applaud all the many cutting-edge doctors who are really looking for the root cause to people's ailments, but if your doctor is just feeding you the party line, it's probably wise for you to find one who's seriously looking for solutions to your health issue. Ask him if it is possible that your problem could be rooted in your acid-base balance, your internal environment, your fluid color, your urine pH-paper color, and see what he says.

CHAPTER 23

BICARB & CANCER

There is a lot of discussion on the internet about bicarbonate, sodium bicarbonate, as a cure for cancer. I am not saying that it does or it doesn't. But I will say, that it is interesting that there is so much opposition against those who believe that bicarbonate can eliminate cancer tumors. Let's just assume that it doesn't work. If it doesn't work, then why would people care so much about shutting it down? If it doesn't work, then you don't have to shoot down the theory, the theory would fail on its own.

If a treatment doesn't work, then it fails and disappears. You don't have to go-after the doctor and take away his license. If it doesn't work, his practice would collapse on its own for lack of success.

The problem is, there are people out there that had tumors and cancer and these ex-cancer patients are the ones making the claims that baking soda cured them.

So the people who think that treating cancer with baking soda is a scam are up against a big problem. The problem being, the patients themselves are claiming that sodium bicarbonate cured them of cancer.

The patients are making the medical claims in favor of bicarbonate.

If you go to www.cancerisafungus.com, that's cancer is a fungus, then click "watch video" in the middle, you will see people who claim that baking soda treatments cured them of cancer. It's interesting. The video is 26 minutes, and if I had cancer I would watch the entire video.

The doctor, Dr. Tullio Simoncini, had his license revoked. I don't see why. I mean, what if it really works? If it really does work to eliminate tumors, then essentially, the Italian government just shut down a doctor for curing cancer. I mean, if people want to go to this guy and he has patients who claim that Dr. Simoncini cured them of their cancer, then isn't that a good thing?

The reader can make up his or her own mind.

The treatment seems pretty radical, inserting catheters into the tumor and then giving yourself baking soda treatments in cycles of 6-days on and 6-days off. But, if I had a tumor, a golfball or a baseball-sized mass, then I would probably take radical treatment.

On the other hand, just keeping my blood slightly alkaline, at its preferred pH of 7.4, and keeping my alkaline stores stocked up, for me is good insurance for cancer prevention, for me personally.

So, I drink one quart of my ABC Water daily to keep my body slightly alkaline, and to keep my alkaline stores stocked up, and this is my personal way of preventing cancer. The readers can do whatever they feel is in the best interests for them.

If I personally had a tumor, the first thing I would do would be to start checking the pH of every one of my urinations and recording them on my weekly chart, and then I would drink ABC Water to keep my urine pH at 7 and 7.2, never letting it drop below 7.

Checking all my urinations is what I should be doing all of the time anyway, but it's a bit time-consuming, so I just go with the one quart of ABC Water per day and another 16 ounces if I perform 30 minutes of heavy physical work or 60 minutes of moderately-hard physical work. Then I spot-check my urine, only checking its pH when I suspect fatigue. This is my daily routine. However, if I had a tumor, I would pay diligent attention to all of my urinations, ensuring that none of them are ever less-than 7 and not higher than 7.2. Just like anything in life, when it becomes a problem, you have to give it more time and attention. That's how I would handle it. The readers are free to decide what would be best for them. So my blood would travel to the tumor and provide slight alkalinity. It's not a radical approach, but more of a soft approach, or mild approach. And I have no idea if it would work, but that's what I would do, because having catheters in my body going to my target organ is a bit risky, in that I would have to keep them sterile since they are entry points to the inside.

It's too bad that science and research are not looking into this baking soda thing. They just negate it and shelve it.

Keep in mind, there are other treatments for cancer that use a lot of freshly-juiced organic vegetables and fruits with no or very little meat. The fruit-and-vegetable juice is basically flooding the body with alkalinity. Plus you get enzymes and color pigments and water and vitamins and minerals.

I have read how it is possible for vegetable juicing to cause a tumor to dissolve so quickly that the cleanup is too much for the liver and kidneys to handle. It's the "Die-Off Effect". The tumor was walled-off, and now it's breaking down, and there is such a mess of toxins being released that the patient feels like he or she is going to die. You have to go slow, so that your liver and kidneys don't get overwhelmed with toxin removal. And if your liver and kidneys aren't all that healthy and functional to begin with, then you have to go even slower.

So if baking soda should ever disappear off the shelves of the supermarket, know that you can always alkalize your body with fruits and vegetables, and ramp up the process by juicing them.

I would sterilize my fruits and vegetables with a lot of clean hot water, cut out any spoiled areas, and buy organic to be sure that I was not getting pesticides, herbicides, fungicides, insecticides, foreign DNA GMOs, sewage-waste fertilizers, and glue added to pesticide spray to make it stick to the plants.

Have you ever been asked to donate a dollar to cancer research as you pay for your groceries at your local supermarket, say, Safeway for example? What kind of research are they doing? Why don't we ever hear about research using bicarbonate to treat tumors? Instead, we just get more sophisticated scans, and treatment procedures, and machines and facilities.

If you made a list of all the treatments that the public believes can cure cancer, I wonder where on that list baking soda would be? I would bet that juicing would be in the top five. What about oxygenation? Actually, if I had a tumor I would go to a hospital here in town that offers 30 minutes in a hyperbaric oxygen chamber. You breathe 100% oxygen for 30 minutes, essentially flooding your body with oxygen. Tumors are anaerobic. They die in the presence of oxygen. Doctor Otto Warburg received a Nobel Prize for his discovery that cancer cannot survive in a high oxygen environment. That means, Oxygen Kills Cancer. A quote from his book says that, "Cancer tissues are acidic, whereas healthy tissues are alkaline." That's interesting.

Another way to get oxygen into your body is Cardiovascular Exercise. I refer to it as Sweat Cardio™. But you would have to be doing it in an area where there is good air and good oxygen, not Central Valley California, since in 2004 we had the worst air quality in the nation. So, go hiking in the mountains where you are surrounded by trees, or move to a northern state such as Washington, Idaho, or Montana, and do outdoor Sweat Cardio three times a day. Washington state has some of the best air I've ever breathed. Move to a rural part of Washington and run a mile before breakfast, run a mile before lunch, and run a mile before dinner. Then buy a trampoline and jump on it. Get as much height as you can on that sucker. Get the tissues, and the lymphatics, and the blood moving, mixing. Stagnant lymph is like having stagnant bowels. Your lymphatic system runs alongside of your blood vessels and is responsible for carrying waste out of the body. It's your sewage system, and you need to keep it moving because it doesn't have a pump like your blood system does. Yoga would do it. Pilates as well. I prefer jumping on a trampoline.

The objective is to get your body to heal itself. Even the doctors and nurses that perform radiation and chemotherapy will tell you that the treatment is part of the process, and that it's expected, or hoped, that your body will do the rest and heal itself.

What if you could skip all that treatment and just get the body to heal itself? That would be my choice. Just get my body to heal itself. Of course, you would have to figure out how to get it to do that.

One time someone asked me what I would do if I had cancer and I told them, freshly-juiced organic fruits and vegetables, sweat cardio before breakfast, lunch, and dinner, hyperbaric oxygen 30 minutes twice a week, and jumping on a trampoline 15 minutes daily. Think outside of your box. God gave you and every one of us the ability to solve problems and to not be helpless little children. Don't limit your choices. Take Control.

I should also have told this person, that if I was doing something bad, I would have to identify it and stop doing it. Specifically, if I smoked I would quit, if I lived in an apartment and was spraying pesticides in my living room, bedroom, and kitchen, I would find a new place to live, if I worked for a microwave-popcorn factory breathing toxic butter flavoring forty hours a week, I would find a different job. The point being, no amount of GOOD will fix the BAD you are being exposed to on a daily basis. You've got to eliminate the bad. Sometimes, just eliminating the bad is all you have to do to get well.™

I used to work at a hospital lab and on the door to the lab was the word "Cancer". "This room contains chemicals known to the State of California to cause cancer." I said to a few of my coworkers, some of them who had worked there for five or more years, that

"We have the word cancer on our door." They never noticed it. Yet it was six inches from their nose every day when they walked in. It's amazing what people don't notice. There was also a list of 19 cancer and birth-defect causing chemicals on the wall next to where people hung their lab coats. Nobody noticed that either. Bizarre. One woman, about 36 years old, died of cervical cancer and left behind the most adorable six- and eight-year-old kids. Sad. Later another coworker announced she had breast cancer and had the double mastectomy. At another hospital where I worked, an employee told me that four people in her department had been diagnosed with cancer in the past year and that the employees were serious about suspecting their workplace as the source. I never heard the outcome, but when the State of California says "This Causes Cancer" they're right, it does.

The government has done its job and told us what causes cancer. People just aren't paying attention. And most people aren't doing much to identify the cancer-causing agents they are putting in their mouths, on their skin, in their lungs, into their tissues. When I press the start button on my microwave I leave the area. A minute later when it beeps, I come back and get my food. Do you keep your cellphone in your pocket next to your body? Is your wireless router for your internet located near your desk or bed? How about your body products? The base chemical for perfumes and colognes is toluene, TNT explosives, Tri Nitro Toluene. However, now that this information has been exposed, companies are trying to clean up their products. There's a maker of cheese slices that now has "No Artificial Preservatives No Artificial Flavoring" printed big on the corner of their product. Oh, like you've been poisoning us with artificial chemicals and flavorings for 40 years and now we're supposed to believe you're the good guys. Good grief.

Not to brag, but when someone I know tells me that they have cancer, I can nearly always see why. Unfortunately, they themselves don't see what causes cancer. The information is available. If you don't know, it's because you haven't looked. Jesus Christ himself said, "and he that seeketh findeth". The answers. The truth about things.

You would do well to know the source of the number one or number two cause of death. The number one cause of death in children is accidents, the number two cause is cancer, leukemia. If you don't get informed for your own sake, you might want to do it for the protection of your children.

I would like to finish this chapter by citing the most amazing testimony of cancer I've ever encountered, Dr. Lorraine Day, www.drday.com. You can read her testimony and history, she is such an inspiration of strength and fearlessness. The photo of her on her homepage is when she was 60 years old, she looks 30. Click in the middle and you will see a photo of her at age 74, she looks 35. But over on the left, click on "Dr. Day's Cancerous Tumor" to see the grapefruit-sized tumor sticking out of her chest. If I had cancer, I would definitely look at what she recommends. Thank you Dr. Day for your courage, books, videos, and common-sense approach to wellness.

Chapter Endnote
"go-after"
My choices were:
You don't have to go after the doctor and take away his license.
(the doctor goes first, then you follow, or, go after)
Whereas "go-after" implies, "chase after" or "hunt after".
You don't have to go-after the doctor and take away his license.
Or I could have written:
You don't have to "investigate someone for possible criminal prosecution" and take away his license. Whew, that's a mouthful.
I hope you were okay with it!

You'll see a hyphenated verb phrase again later on, (give-in).

CHAPTER 24

BICARB & HYPERTENSION

So, I was in the kitchen one day making the NCD Taco Salad™ recipe and I decided I was going to switch from canned kidney beans to dried kidney beans. Remembering BPA for a minute, they also discovered BPA being used to line canned foods, and that waxy shiny coating on cash register tapes, that's also bisphenol A. My philosophy for making a meal and designing a new recipe is, start with some canned, packaged, or frozen food, if you need to, to make the recipe taste good, then improve the recipe by making it yourself from scratch. But it doesn't always work, as my recent attempts at making Alfredo Sauce wasn't as good as the one I buy at Trader Joe's in the glass jar. The linings of glass food items are not coated with BPA, and this is another reason to make glass your first choice in the kitchen.

So back to the kidney beans, the first batch just would not soften, even after boiling them for two hours and letting them sit overnight. The second batch wasn't any better, even though I did a presoak and added salt to the water. That's when I turned to the internet for help.

One lady said her beans would not soften and then her husband came along and added the diced tomatoes to them. She stated that the acid from the tomato juice would make it impossible for the beans to soften. Others said that you have to add baking soda to the water, or, scientifically speaking, raise the pH of the water, if you have hard tap water, which I do, it's 13 according to my local water company.

Hm.

So my bean problem was not due to insufficient heating, it wasn't that my beans were stale, as I had just purchased them from the store and the best-by date was good, and it wasn't that I never added salt to the water. The beans weren't softening because my soaking-water was acidic and not alkaline. I needed to add a water "softener". That's interesting.

Well, I added baking soda to the soak water, cooked my beans, and voila, they were soft. In fact, the first batch came out too soft, so I had to cut back on the cooking time.

So, the acid from the tomato juice hardens and the bicarbonate from the baking soda softens.

Then it occurred to me in a flash. What if high blood pressure, hypertension, that so many people these days are experiencing, is caused by their body being too acidic? What if, by alkalizing the body you could lower your blood pressure?

If I made that claim I would go to jail, so I am not making that claim, or any other claim. This is simply my personal experience, and based on my personal experience, I personally believe that hypertension can be lowered by shifting the balance of acid alkaline towards the direction of alkaline. The three ways to do this are, as we've already discussed, change your diet by eating more fruits and vegetables and less animal protein, or supplement with bicarbonate, or a little of both, a combination of the two.

That acidic blood makes vessel walls tighten, and that alkaline blood makes vessel walls soften, just makes sense to me.

There are lots of variables and reasons for high blood pressure, although, the medical profession will admit they don't know what the cause or reasons are for ESSENTIAL hypertension, so I am not saying that increasing your alkalinity will work for you. But what if it worked for 10% of the hypertensive patients, or 30% or 50% of all those with hypertension? Sixty-five million of our fellow Americans have hypertension. So if half of them were hypertensive due to acidosis, that would be 32,500,000 people who could potentially correct their blood pressure by supplementing with bicarbonate.

And what about that word "Essential", as though it's an essential part of life, like an essential fatty acid or essential vitamins and minerals. As though everyone has to have it, so by making it COMMON it becomes NORMAL. Cancer is becoming like that, in that they are saying that by such-and-such a date that almost everyone will have had cancer at some point during their lifetime. I'm surprised they don't call it "Essential Cancer". "Oh, we don't know what causes it, everyone has it, don't feel bad, there's nothing you can do, just come with me and I'll get you started on your radiation treatments." Don't let other people try to persuade you that something that's ABNORMAL is NORMAL.

Did you know that the medical profession was once found guilty of trying to eliminate the chiropractic profession? Imagine if you had been a chiropractor during the 1980s, and you and your colleagues are under attack by the physicians and surgeons to have your entire profession eliminated. Fortunately for chiropractors, and the public, they fought back and won, even though they were much smaller in power than the American Medical Association. By attempting to eliminate the competition, you are attempting to create a monopoly, whereby your group is the only choice. Isn't the founding principle of a "Free Market Economy" that everyone gets to play? Kudos to the justice system for standing against the medical profession and allowing chiropractors their profession.

My dictionary defines "Essential" as "Necessary". So I ask you, mister medical profession, why did you choose the word "essential" or necessary for hypertension? Are you trying to get the public to believe that it's just NORMAL, just a part of life?

There being no treatment for getting rid of it, and you are told that you will take these pills for the rest of your life.

Here's where, not allowing others to think for you could possibly save you a lot of grief and money. Where wisdom for the game of life may keep you from having an operation and losing most of your monopoly assets, if you have a clue.

My personal belief, that acid can increase your blood pressure and alkalizing can lower it, as with the kidney beans and the alkaline water, isn't enough to make my experience appear on the nightly news and become mainstream. It would require large crossover double-blind placebo-controlled studies, but, like the attempt at eliminating chiropractors, I don't think this study will be performed anytime soon.

Healthcare makes up 15% of the total economy. Now I am not suggesting or implying anything, but just suppose a solution for everyone's problems was to happen overnight, a panacea if you will. No more sickness or disease or chronic anything. There would be a shift in spending dollars from healthcare to other places, or you could invest the money you were no longer spending on healthcare. Do you think God intended for us to have so many health problems, and hundreds and hundreds of disease names, more and more disease names every year? I don't believe he did. I believe we do it to ourselves.

The A aspect of this book pertains to supplementing with alkalinity due to being alkaline deficient, due to an imbalance of diet, too much meat and protein, and not enough fruits and vegetables. If that weren't bad enough, we create additional acid in our bodies by working out and exercising, taking medications, pollution, and the whole gamut of toxic emotions, negative thinking, and bad memories. Even if you did eat 3-5 fruits and vegetables a day, you would still likely come up short on alkalinity. To me this seems so obviously the cause of so many problems, but no popular mainstream book, no mainstream TV program, no celebrity, no one at all is discussing it. Except Here.

ALKALINE DEFICIENCY™ – you heard it here first.

Now it may be that it is just too complicated for the average person, but I have more faith and belief in the average everyday person. If a diabetic patient knows that his or her hemoglobin A1c needs to be less-than 6, and a cancer patient knows how to say "adenocarcinoma", then learning to check your urine pH and aiming it at 7 is no big deal. For those interested, I just came back from the restroom and using my 0-13 pH strip, the color was halfway between 6 and 7, so approximately 6.5. Three sips of ABC Water, just to make sure that my next one is closer to 7 and not closer to 6, and that's it. It's not hard once you start doing it. As a matter of fact, with the system I have outlined here, it will be very easy for you to do. The hard part will just be the initial setup, but if you review the Strategy Chapter it's very do-able. Until now, there has never, that I am aware of, been a complete and comprehensive step-by-step guide for taking control of your acid alkaline status, and raising your alkalinity safely, properly, and responsibly.

I came across another way that reduced my blood pressure problem. It's magnesium. Now this is no secret to many of you. In my case, I had been taking a lot of coral calcium supplements after I discovered that the phosphoric acid in the pepsi-cola I was addicted to was leaching calcium from my bones, and my high coral calcium intake made my body become low on magnesium, as calcium and magnesium compete with each other for absorption in the colon. Add to that a lot of sweat cardio, where you lose electrolytes, along with magnesium, and within a few months, I determined that I was low on mag.

Magnesium and calcium have an effect on vessel walls in much the same way as pH. Calcium tenses, and magnesium relaxes, or softens. That is why too much calcium makes you calcium dominant, causing vessel wall tenseness, exhibited by high blood pressure. Conversely, magnesium counteracts the effects of calcium, causing vessel walls to relax and soften, with a subsequent lowering of blood pressure.

Think of calcium as having the same effect in your body as acidosis, tensing, and think of magnesium as doing the same thing as alkalizing, softening. There is nothing wrong with calcium, just as there is nothing wrong with acid production, you simply have to be sure to balance calcium with sufficient magnesium, and balance acidity with sufficient alkalinity.

I purchased magnesium at www.nutrabio.com, that's Nutra Bio, (888) 688-7224.   You will notice they have the words "Pure Supplements" under their name. I do believe they are pure, and this is why I buy from them, but, purity is now popular, and the original supplement company that began the purity trend, making purity their number-one priority and the foundation of their company, was Dr. Clark Store. When you view a product at Nutra Bio, click on the "Quality" tab and you will see a list, kosher, vegetarian, hypoallergenic, non-GMO, gluten free, rBST, fillers, excipients, GMP, and label disclosure. This is excellent! Thank you Nutra Bio. Disclosure Disclosure Disclosure. This company hides nothing. The customer should feel confident buying from a company like this. I don't use protein powder, but I think I am going to buy a container of their Whey Protein Concentrate. Each serving is 25g of protein, so about the same as a 4oz chicken breast, and you get 69 servings for $51, that works out to about $0.74 for a "chicken breast" amount of protein powder.

If you look at the label for the Whey Protein ISOLATE, which is $62, higher in price because it has 10% more protein than the Concentrate, and no fat, and less carbs, if you scroll down you will see their "Full Label Disclosure" and under "other ingredients" they boast the words "Absolutely None". Both of these products are 100% whey protein, from dairy, with no added anything. It's fantastic. Especially when you compare their label to other brands.

So click on the "minerals" tab at the top, then click on Magnesium Chelate. I bought the Magnesium Chelate 500g item #24141, it's $26. Two of their spoon "scoops" equals 400mg of magnesium. This is not the exact product I purchased, and unfortunately, the percent of the magnesium is now half of what my label says, unless they made a labeling error and they really mean one scoop is 400mg of mag, rather than two scoops being 400mg of mag. My label says one scoop, 1143mg, provides 400mg of elemental magnesium, and their current product label says two scoops, 2222mg provides 400mg of magnesium. Hm. Well, the one bad thing about this company, and they do elude to it on their website, is that they change labels from time to time, perhaps it has something to do with a certain batch or lot number. None-the-less, here's where I bought magnesium powder.

In the beginning I took 500mg of magnesium with my breakfast meal, just sprinkle it on top of whatever you are having, and 500mg with my dinner meal. Later, I dropped it to once a day. Currently I just have a 500mg spoonful sporadically, or daily if I feel my blood pressure has gone up, which can happen if I have more than five grams of "salt" in one day. The NCD Beef Dip™ recipe is delicious, but for the au-jus I use Worcestershire sauce diluted with water. It tastes perfect, just like you would get at a restaurant, but one of the ingredients on the Worcester bottle is Natural Flavorings, and don't be fooled by the word "Natural" as it could be any number of things, including chemicals, and including MSG, monosodium glutamate.

It would be nice if Lea & Perrins would DISCLOSE what exactly is in that "Natural Flavoring" they are using. Did you know that that flavor enhancer "Accent" in the white-and-red cardboard cylinder-shaped container in the seasoning aisle, did you know that that product is 100% Monosodium Glutamate? Flavor should come from your food, not from chemical flavoring enhancers. And then people wonder why they are addicted to certain foods. You don't think restaurants know how to get you to come back?

I would like to commend the Heinz corporation for their yellow mustard label, which no longer lists "natural flavoring" but instead lists just five simple foods, vinegar, mustard seed, salt, turmeric, and paprika. Thank you Heinz for revising your food label and product to list ingredients that I can recognize, I don't need a PhD in chemistry, nor do I have to search government websites for what constitutes an ingredient like "natural flavoring".

So it is that I believe, that acid has a tensing effect on blood vessels like calcium does, and alkalinity softens and relaxes blood vessels like magnesium does.

For those of you who have very high blood pressure and are desperate for something that will help, a fast effective blood-pressure dropper, in my experience, is an Epsom Salt Bath. Epsom salt is magnesium sulfate. I bought mine at the "99 Cents Store" and it says on the front, Magnesium Sulfate U.S.P., so it's pharmaceutical grade, the best grade you can buy. Wow. It comes in a 2lb 907g one-quart container, and I use half the container, about 2 cups, in a full bathtub of water. Soak in it for 45 minutes, keeping as much of your skin submerged under the water as possible. It is important to maintain the water at about 100°F or 38°C so that the pores of the skin open and absorb the magnesium. A tepid bath won't do the trick, your skin needs to be a little pink. I suggest using a thermometer so you don't overdo it with the hot water. If it's too hot, you won't be able to stay in it for more than a few minutes, whereas 100° is hot enough to open your pores, yet cool enough to allow you to soak for 45 minutes. If you shorten the incubation time to less-than 45 minutes, you'll get less of an effect. In my experience it dropped my blood pressure to lows that I've never seen before.

Lastly, a discussion of sodium and salt is needed as many people are confused. Sodium, in its free ionic form, Na+, is good and needed. We love free sodium. Free sodium helps keep our body alkaline by grabbing our precious bicarbonate from the urine and pulling it back into the body. Sodium-chloride is tablesalt and is not the same as free sodium, tablesalt is a sodium attached to a chloride. When you eat tablesalt, the sodium and the chloride break apart, but then the blood sees too much chloride and signals the body to eliminate it, so the chloride binds to the sodium and out it goes in the urine. So, you eat sodium-chloride, tablesalt, and that same sodium-chloride gets eliminated, without gaining any free sodium in the process.

Or, if sodium-chloride elimination is slowed down because of a steady flow of tablesalt intake from the diet, then the blood becomes high in free sodium and free chloride. As long as the chloride is there, the sodium has to be there to balance it out. If you could get rid of the chloride in the bloodstream, then the sodium could leave and go do its other jobs in the tissues. It's the chloride that's evil. The chloride is holding sodium hostage in the bloodstream. So now, water enters the blood vessel to dilute the sodium concentration. And there you have your high blood pressure.

The CHLORIDE is holding the sodium HOSTAGE in the bloodstream. Sodium is the good guy. It's the chloride that's bad. This is why apple cider vinegar is considered an alkalizer, even though it's an acid, acetic acid. A good-quality ACV should contain a lot of the minerals from the apples, minerals like calcium and magnesium, that are positively charged and can lower chloride levels. Less chloride means sodium is free to leave the bloodstream and go do its job elsewhere in the body. Apples also contain sodium malate. The malate gets burned as fuel and leaves behind free sodium. Plant salt is the opposite of tablesalt. But they just put all salts under one heading and say "salt is bad". The more plant sodium you can get in your diet the better.

They don't tell you the whole story, and that is this. The high blood pressure is caused by too much water in the blood vessel. The extra water is there because of the sodium. And the sodium is there because of the chloride. That's the part they don't tell you. That last step tells you who the real culprit is, and that culprit is the CHLORIDE, tablesalt. And chlorinated drinking-water.

Sodium-Chloride is a hydrator. But high blood pressure, in the initial stages, is a state of overhydration, ballooned up blood vessels from too much chloride consumption. Do you find it interesting that nobody on TV or that any of the well-known health celebrity personalities ever mentions chloride?

Instead they just keep leading us astray by saying "salt". It's not salt, it's tablesalt, and chemical salts, and it's not sodium, it's chloride, and glutamate.

We see the same thing regarding cholesterol. They say that high blood cholesterol levels increase the risk of heart disease. Why do they say this?   Because cholesterol is found in plaque, and eventually that plaque buildup can shut off the blood flow through the vessel, occlusion. But why is your body making plaque? Your body's not stupid, everything it does, it does for a reason. What's the reason? Well, we now know it's due to inflammation of the vessel walls.   So, what's causing the vessel walls to be inflamed? Well, they won't say because they don't want to point fingers. We already discussed how chlorine tablets thicken the vessel walls, so chlorine, and its sister fluorine/fluoride, and its other sister bromine/bromide, found in baked goods from brominated flour, and in Mountain Dew soda pop from brominated vegetable oil, are inflammatory molecules, along with many other free radicals and toxins we put into our bodies unaware of what we are doing to ourselves. Someone once said, we dig our graves one mouthful at a time. There's wisdom in that, if you will take heed. So back to the cholesterol, it can best be explained like this. Just because you find firemen at the scene of a fire, that doesn't mean they're the bad guys. They're there to put out the fire of inflammation in the wall of the blood vessel. The same is true for cholesterol. If your body hadn't taken cholesterol and repaired the vessel wall, your vessel would have leaked or hemorrhaged. That cholesterol plaque just saved the person's life. That's exactly how the body responds. The body compensates to keep you alive. Your SYMPTOMS are SIGNS of COMPENSATION for something you are doing wrong.

Your   SYMPTOMS   are   SIGNS   of   COMPENSATION   for something you are doing wrong.™

There are doctors that are going against the establishment and saying that, "High cholesterol has very little to do with increasing your risk of heart disease." This is true. How courageous these doctors are as they could potentially bring an end to the over-emphasized blood tests for cholesterol, and an end to prescribing statins to lower cholesterol. These courageous doctors go on to say that, "People are waking up to the truth." You my friend would do well to do the same.

So, stop consuming CHLORIDE and your blood pressure goes down.

Now, unrefined seasalt has sodium-chloride, but it also has the positively charged minerals that will lower chloride levels. This is why Celtic and Himalayan salts are better because of the calcium, magnesium, zinc, copper, iron, and other minerals they contain.

You want to eat foods that supply free sodium, Na+, not foods that contain sodium-chloride. Surely you've heard of the Three White Foods everyone should avoid; Refined White Flour, which is long chains of fast sugar, high glycemic; Refined White Sugar, which has such a stimulating effect that it has been compared to street drugs, and in fact, in the movies the detective opens the bag and tastes the white powder to see if it's cocaine or sugar; and Refined White Salt, mineral-depleted 100% sodium-chloride. So, refined refined refined. There we have man tampering with the food supply again, when God didn't design it that way. Choose God's design.

The other sodium product that is not allowed on the NCD™ plan is sodium attached to an amino acid, like sodium glutamate, aka, monosodium glutamate MSG. This is another highly stimulating compound that will totally shoot my blood pressure up by 40-50 points if I consume a lot of it in one day, or a moderate amount over several days, or a lesser amount over several weeks. MSG should never be consumed. And the public is aware of this because some chinese-food restaurants and food manufacturers have put claims on their products that they do not use MSG. Canned soups are notorious for containing MSG, and as stated earlier, any time you see the word "FLAVORING" regardless of whether it says natural in front of it, flavoring can be just about anything, including MSG. When you see "flavoring", put the word CHEMICAL in front of it, as that's what it is.

"SPICES" on a food label is another one to be aware of. If you trust the company, then spices might just be spices, but if the company also sells foods with high-fructose corn syrup, then in my opinion, you can assume that they will throw MSG or some other laboratory-designed chemical in there and call it "spices". The biological harm of HFCS is well established so any food company that uses it in any of their products is, in my opinion, untrustworthy and should therefore be boycotted.

So free sodium is what you want, and this can be obtained from plants; fruits and vegetables, nuts and seeds, beans and legumes. They contain sodium attached to carbohydrates, and when these break apart, the carbohydrate portion gets burned as fuel and the sodium is free to go off and do its important work elsewhere.

Sodium bicarbonate then, our baking soda, and potassium bicarbonate, are in the same category as plant sodium, in that, they contain no chloride. The **sodium** separates from the bicarbonate and then goes to the kidneys to retrieve bicarbonate that is being used to remove hydrogen ions (acid), and the **free bicarbonate** is used to directly neutralize hydrogen ions (acid). So, Baking Soda is a DOUBLE ALKALIZER. It dissociates into free sodium and free bicarbonate, both of which function to create and alkaline internal environment.

Now the potassium bicarbonate is added to the ABC Water™ recipe formulation so that you don't become sodium dominant. And because fruits and vegetables are loaded with potassium, the ABC Water functions as a substitute for fruits and vegetables. Remembering that the real thing should always be your first choice for alkalinity, and that ABC Water fills in the gap for your current and prior history of not getting enough plant foods in your diet, the solution to our modern-day diet and lifestyles, in my opinion.

Lastly, I said chloride was evil, but that was with regard to blood pressure and sodium retention. Chloride is needed in the body to make hydrochloric acid, secreted by the stomach when we eat protein. We need HCl to digest the protein in our meal, but there is no shortage of chloride in our bodies or our diets, just like we need phosphorus in our bodies but there is no shortage of phosphorus either. On the contrary, chlorinated water and phosphate fertilizers provide more than enough of these two nutrients.

In conclusion, when backtracking to the root cause of hypertension, and the root cause of arterial plaque, the backtracking stops one step short. This is done to prevent finger-pointing, and no one wants to point fingers at the root problems when money is being made on the front-end. This is basic free-market economics, and we are all a part of it. Your job is to navigate your way through life, seeking the truth that you will surely find, per Jesus Christ's personally guaranteed word, and use that truth to make wise choices, which is what King Solomon wanted even more than gold and silver. Sodium is not the bad guy, it's chloride. What causes high chloride in the body, chlorinated water, and white refined mineral-depleted sodium-chloride salt. Chemical salts are ten-times worse than chloride salts, therefore, NO MSG EVER, NO NATURAL FLAVORING EVER, and NO "SPICES". And if you are drinking chlorinated water straight from the tap, use a charcoal filter, or switch to reverse osmosis.

Good sodium is free sodium, and it's obtained from eating plants, unrefined salts, or it can be supplemented by taking baking soda when dietary consumption of plants and unrefined salts is lacking. Fruits and vegetables are also where most of our dietary potassium comes from, so a sodium potassium "baking soda" is ideal. Baking soda also contains another plant nutrient, bicarbonate, the "janitor" of the body who works nonstop mopping up the mess (the acid).

The statements in this chapter and throughout this entire publication are based on the author's personal experience, knowledge, understanding, and conclusions regarding this understanding, and as stated throughout this book, this information is for informational purposes only and no claims are being made as to the treatment of hypertension or any other medical condition. The reader is a free agent and is free to decide what is in his or her best interests and free to act according to those best interests.

CHAPTER 25

B17

There is one other B vitamin worth mentioning, and that is Vitamin B17, also known as Laetrile, and Amygdalin. You'll be hard-pressed to find this vitamin sold in stores as the FDA banned it back in the 1980s, after some books were published saying that B17, laetrile, helped your body combat cancer.

Only the FDA can make claims that a nutrient can do something. Although we are all entitled to our own opinions and our own thinking under the freedoms and principles of free speech that all developed nations uphold, there is no law that says that anyone HAS to believe what the FDA says. And it is interesting to note how many drugs the FDA approves and then later they get pulled off the market, so clearly, if you have to UNapprove something a few years later, then you made an error in the beginning. I am not bashing the FDA as they are under a lot of pressure to do and to not do certain things, but as an adult, you have to decide what you are going to believe as you journey your way through life.

For me, I figure, since a vitamin is defined as a biological nutrient that the body cannot make, then we have to get it from our diets. But what if you're not getting enough? What if your diet over the past ten years hasn't supplied you with any significant B17? We never hear about it. And yet it exists.

Apparently, liver and organ meats contain a lot of vitamins and minerals, but I haven't eaten liver since I was a teenager in the late 1970s living at home and my mom used to make liver and onions once every few months. For this reason, I started buying Apricot Kernels. They are high in B17, and there are a lot of people who eat them solely for this reason. So here's what you can do.

Funny, I just printed something from the internet about B17, and my internet connection just went down. Hm. Is there something about B17 that someone just doesn't want us to know?

Go to www.SwansonVitamins.com, type "raw apricot kernels" in the search-box, and there you will see Swanson's Certified Organic Raw Apricot Kernels, 12oz 340g for $12.99. I was able to take advantage of one of their many promo offers, purchasing two bags with 10% off and free shipping. This website has hundreds of products, some pure, some have additives, so I only purchase certain items here, but they have some excellent products at fair prices. So buy two bags, and start eating them. I love them. They're delicious. In fact, the thought occurred to me that the REASON why I am eating so many and my body still wants more, is that MAYBE I'M DEFICIENT IN B17. My body is saying, "Finally! I've been looking for some B17 for the past ten years and there's been none available." Chomp chomp chomp.

There is a warning on the package that says not to eat more than eight kernels per day, and the information I read says that you may experience a headache or dizziness if you eat too many at one time. It also says that vitamin B17 contains a CN– cyanide molecule, but that so does vitamin B12, as well as chickpeas and strawberries. Plant cyanide, or plant fluoride, is different from industrial fluoride, or laboratory cyanide.

When the bags arrived in the mail, I divided one 12oz package into six servings of two ounces each, and I vacuum sealed five servings and then placed the remaining 2oz in a small glass jar with screw cap (the 2oz glass jar purchased at sks-bottle.com). I eat a few kernels every so often, and then at the start of a new month I open a new 2oz bag. This works out to 2oz x 12 months, or 24oz a year, or two of Swanson's bags per year.   I figure this is enough to supply me with vitamin B17.

I store the 2oz vacuum-sealed bags of my apricot kernels in a brown-paper bag to protect them from oxidation by light, and store the brown bag in the refrigerator to prevent oxidation from heat, and the vacuum sealing has removed all the air so they're protected from oxidation by oxygen.

The original bags had a best-by date of about 30 months from the date I received them, and the literature says the kernels are good 4 months at room temperature or 12 months in the refrigerator, so I wouldn't buy more than two bags at a time.

Finally, there's that word, Amygdalin, Amygdalin, Amygdalin, where have I heard this word before?   Oh, Amygdala, those two almond-shaped glands located near the base of the brain.   Now, amygdalin B17, is not the same spelling as amygdala, but it is interesting that they are similarly spelled words.   Does this area of the brain, the amygdala, have a high concentration or some dependent relationship with amygdalin, vitamin B17?   Does the fear emotion cause the amygdala to use up vitamin B17, resulting in low amygdalin levels?   These are good questions.   Anyway, like anything else related to taking care of your health, if you feel you need to get approval from your doctor before you begin eating apricot kernels, then by all means do so.   This discussion was for informational purposes only.

CHAPTER 26

BODY BUILDERS

This chapter addresses bodybuilders, athletes, and exercise enthusiasts, because, unlike people who don't exercise, these people produce post-workout acid.

Surely we've all read, or may know someone who, "died of a heart attack while playing tennis" "died during a workout" "collapsed during practice and never recovered" or the one I was recently told about by a colleague of mine, "He was a fitness trainer and he had a heart attack, fell into the pool, and died in his early 40s." This is not to scare you, but to have you seriously consider your acid alkaline status before exercising. This is one reason people are told to check with their doctor before beginning an exercise program.

The acid produced from exercise, if not neutralized and eliminated, can deplete alkaline stores. When this happens, the body chokes, like how you would choke for air when you hold your breath, but in this case the body is choking for alkalinity. If there's none available, you end up with these statistics of people dying during or after their workout.

We all want to push our limits when performing our sport, it's that drive in us to be better, run further, jump higher, lift heavier. It's similar to when you injure a bodypart, you didn't have enough strength to do it and you went for it anyway, and something gave way. So, the athlete keeps working out, doing drills, running, throwing, jumping, and ignoring the signals that the body is saying, "Hey, I'm feeling exhausted." Exercise shouldn't take you to exhaustion. There should always be something left, some energy remaining. Some fitness advisors tell their clients that they have to "give 100% and leave everything on the gym floor", essentially walking out of the gym on empty.

As you WALK out the door of the gym, your cardiovascular system has returned to normal, but your muscles are still cooking up acid, acid that was going out the lungs on a real-time basis when you were breathing hard, but is now just piling up inside your body. This is the concept behind the "cool-down" ending of a workout. But for a weightlifting workout, there isn't a lot of cardio, so there's not a lot of heavy breathing, so there's not a lot of acid escaping through the lungs. But, there is A LOT of acid being produced in the muscles. So what happens? Two hours later, you're fried, crashed, and eating everything in sight to get your energy back up. Metabolic acidosis is setting in.

INSTEAD OF OVEREATING, JUST ALKALIZE™.

If your alkaline reserves are already depleted, you are at risk and in a dangerous physiological state. Your cardiovascular system is turned down to low, your muscles are pumped and metabolically active, and your alkaline reserves are depleted.

Quick, I've got to drink my protein shake, eat my chicken, or scarf down my tuna.

When what you should be doing is giving your body, Anti-Acid, Anti-Stress, and Anti-Oxidant, ABC Water™, alkalinity, vitamin B, vitamin C, and hydration.

Don't freak out because you missed your post-workout anabolic window by 15 minutes. The theory behind this is that blood is flowing at its maximum after a workout, but your blood flows every second of every day, so your shake will get to your muscles, don't worry.

I find that anabolism kicks in any time I feel rested, healthy, and upbeat. Then I eat a meal with protein fats and carbs, and boom!, my muscles just start expanding. You really do want the "Incredible Hulk" effect, where his shirt splits and his body muscles expand and grow. This is anabolism. Your goal is to have this occur as often as possible during the hours and days after your workout, the period of time when your muscles regrow bigger than they were before, aka, the recovery period. This state requires an alkaline internal environment. Your urine pH is your best indicator of this.

You can get an anabolic effect just from eating a meal, without working out. I call this the "Sirloin Steak Effect". Grill yourself some steak or bake some prime rib in the oven and Boom! Your muscles pump up as if you had just spent 45 minutes in the gym.

A muscle pump, or anabolic effect, can happen at any time, not just within 30 minutes after a workout. You should be eating balanced high-nutrient meals all day long, so as to feed your muscles on a constant 3 hour basis, or 2, 2.5, or every 4 hours, depending on what your objective is, bulk, maintain, or cut.

After a workout, your body is going to be spending the next 24 or 48 or 72 hours repairing and recovering, so you had better be supplying it with regular intervals of macro-balanced high nutrient-rich meals. The Number Crunch Diet™ is precisely designed for the bodybuilder and athlete, in that, the recipes are macro balanced, the calories of the meals are all set to 500, making calorie tracking super easy, in that you count calories by counting Pre-Counted Meals™. The post-workout shake is fine, but the biggest factors contributing to your growth are the 6 or 12 or 18 meals you will be eating every 2.5 hours during the next 1 to 2 to 3 days after your workout. IT'S THESE MEALS that have the potential to generate an anabolic effect.

Your meals are fueling your growth and recovery.™

Your MEALS are FUELING your GROWTH and RECOVERY.

Your post-workout shake is just one meal. What have you got planned or prepared in your refrigerator for your next 11 or 17 meals over the next 2 to 3 days?

Poor nutrition after a workout means poor recovery, poor muscle growth, and poor results, and then you give up, or worse, you turn to steroids to get some results. In fact, you may actually end up with smaller muscles over time because you keep breaking them down during your workouts, yet not supplying them with adequate nutrition to rebuild. Or, if you do get results by eating low-quality food, fastfood, packaged and processed food, it may just be that you have youth hormones on your side. But what are you going to do in your 40s and 50s when your youth hormones are missing-in-action and you never took the time in your 20s and 30s to learn how to make your own meals and build a recipe repertoire?

JPM's Number Crunch Diet™ has everything you need, and a variety of meals to choose from.

The faster you recover the sooner you can work out again, repeating the cycle of muscle challenge, muscle breakdown, muscle buildup. This is the premise behind steroids. They artificially pump you back up so you can be back in the gym lifting more and heavier in one to two days. But that's cheating. Surely you recall that world-famous cyclist who was stripped of all seven of his Tour de France first-place titles for cheating. But he's by no means the only one. Many many pro and nonprofessional athletes have used performance-enhancing drugs. Don't be a cheater. Eat the Number Crunch Diet Performance-Enhancing Meals instead.

Along with the NCD meals used to support recovery, try drinking ABC Water and keeping your urine pH at 7 as a second way to speed recovery.™

Nip that acidosis in the bud, and get your body back to its healthy alkaline state ASAP. You'll be feeling better, have more energy, and be finding yourself back in the gym in record time. You heard it here first.

CHAPTER 27

pH & Stones

Another reason for keeping your urine pH at exactly 7 is for the prevention of crystals and stone formations, aka, renal calculi. Similar to the calculi your dental hygienist removes, these mineral salts, or plaques, are not what you want to have occur. Crystals are more likely to occur in an acidic urine, with 75% of all kidney stones being composed of calcium oxalate crystals.

Think about your dietary habits for a moment.

In my early days, I worked as a waiter and bartender at a restaurant on Beverly Drive in Beverly Hills. The first thing I noticed was, that approximately half the customers ordered a 32oz glass of iced tea, that's 4 cups of tea, and then they proceeded to sweeten it with pink, yellow, and blue packets of artificial sweetener. This just goes to prove, you can have money, but not wisdom, at least not as far as diet and health are concerned.

Tea is loaded with oxalates. Oxalates are most likely to be seen in an acidic urine. They are known to be found occasionally in a pH neutral urine, and also found rarely in an alkaline urine. But 9 out of 10 times oxalates will be found in an acidic urine. This means that you can avoid the creation of kidney stones by two-thirds, (75% x 9/10), just by keeping your urine pH out of the acidic zone.

The crystal that forms when you drink tea is called Calcium

Oxalate. The oxalate from the tea, binds to the calcium from the blood or bones, and shows up in the urine. This creates the potential for renal-calculi formation in the kidneys, as well as osteoporosis in the bones. Just like how water pulls soft-plastic chemicals from the interior surface of plastic water bottles, oxalates pull calcium out of the bones.

The same is true for colas. These junk-food beverages contain zero nutrition. To make them worse, they contain harmful health-damaging ingredients. They are Anti-Nutrition. Nothing good, and all bad. Some medical professionals will say that the reason they are bad is because they are high in sodium. Read the label. There's very little sodium listed. What they are loaded with is phosphoric acid, phosphates. I am not going to tell you that they are loaded with high-fructose corn syrup, because you should already know this. I regard soft drinks as poisons. And yes, I am as guilty as most people are for having consumed them, although, there are people who have never consumed a soft drink ever in their entire lives. Their inner wisdom was telling them "don't" "it's not good". I had that inner wisdom when it came to margarine, but I didn't see the harm of soda pop, or maybe I neglected to see it because something in me was hooked on them. I see it now though.

Phosphates bind calcium to form calcium phosphate crystals, and these crystals like to form in an alkaline pH. So, if your urine pH is higher than 7, you risk having calcium-phosphate crystal formation occurring, especially if you are a cola drinker. Although these crystals are not commonly seen, due to the fact that very few people have an alkaline urine, none-the-less, an overabundance of phosphate in the diet removes calcium from the bones, and this is an undeniable fact that you will never hear on television, because no one will point fingers at the source.

So, the two most common beverages available in eating establishments and vending machines, colas and tea, have the potential to produce crystals and stones at both ends of the pH scale, acid and alkaline. For me, the safest place is neutral. A neutral pH of 7.   So pick your poison, colas or teas, you lose calcium either way.

Well what about green tea you ask, we hear a lot about green tea being recommended as good for you.   The NCD plan says no to caffeine, and this includes caffeinated teas.   There are other places where you can get your antioxidants and flavonoids from without the stimulation of caffeine, like in fruits and vegetables.   The same thing applies to red wine.   You can get resveratrol and polyphenols from grapes, grape juice, or raisins, as well as other fruits and vegetables, without consuming ethanol, an alternative gasoline source that is toxic to your liver.   So here's your liver busy working and cleaning things up, and then you slam on the brakes with a glass of wine.   Plus alcohol dehydrates you and dehydration causes aging.   A lot of what nurses do is simple, and expensive, hydration.

The NCD forbids caffeine and alcohol.   Try to function and get the energy you need without stimulants, try the ABC Water.   Try to relax and purge stress and anxiety without alcohol, try the ABC Water.

The NCD does have a recipe that includes red wine as the beverage, and it's served in a fancy wine glass, but the volume of wine with the meal is 30 grams, or one fluid ounce.   You don't need 6-8 ounces of wine to enjoy your dinner and have a good time.   One ounce of wine sipped on slowly is adequate.   Any more than one ounce means that your motive has switched from enjoying dinner, to getting a buzz and escaping your problems for a while.   This is fruitless.   You will never escape your problems and stresses.   When the alcohol wears off, there will be your problems again staring you right in the face.   But now you're in a weaker state and less able to deal with them.   So what do you do?   You escape again.   Alcohol leads to alcoholism.   Just don't go there.

The NCD doesn't allow "Moderation".   Moderation, in my opinion, is kind of middle-of-the-road, halfway there already.   The NCD says "Moderation is Too Much".™   Instead, you can have certain foods Occasionally or Rarely.   The NCD recipes RARELY have HFCS and Natural Flavorings, and OCCASIONALLY have caffeine, or theobromine (caffeine's cousin found in cocoa), in the form of a small amount of dark chocolate.   Nescafé makes decaffeinated coffee and if you add a little bit to milk, you can fool yourself into thinking you're drinking a venti mocha whatever.

This technique of having something similar, but without the addictive ingredients, allows a person to break free of their addiction to certain beverages or foods. The NCD program has ways to break food addictions so stay tuned!

In conclusion, avoid oxalates found in teas, and phosphates found in colas, as these products are simply bottled and processed manufactured formulations. If that weren't bad enough, both teas and colas leach calcium out of the body resulting in calcium-oxalate and calcium-phosphate crystals respectively.   A neutral urine pH of 7, the same as that of plain water, is your safest bet to avoid crystal and renal-calculi formation. Any argument that colas and teas have nothing to do with kidney stones and crystal formation, is simply nonsense.

Chapter Endnote

There are two camps when it comes to hyphenating fractions. One group says, do not hyphenate if the denominator functions as a noun, only hyphenate if the fraction functions as an adjective. The other group says you should hyphenate all fractions regardless. I decided to go with the second camp, since, as a number, it's 2 slash 3, then as a written word it makes more sense to be two hyphen three.   Also, as a noun, "two" is not modifying "thirds", the fraction is a unit, "two-thirds". While we're on the subject of math, if you see "~", read the word "about" or "approximately", ~10, about ten.

CHAPTER 28

pH & Inflammation

I've used the word "urine" several dozen times. Some of you may thinking, "that's gross". Well, if your urine is gross, you've got a medical problem. Your urine should be sterile, clear, yellow, and pH neutral. A healthy urine is just plain water with a few organic and inorganic compounds. Nothing gross about it.

But what's key is, this fluid was just part of your blood. Blood that just circulated around your entire body from head to toe. This blood enters your kidneys, the kidneys filter it and make urine, and you now have an opportunity to see what's happening throughout your body at the level of pH. I've referred to pH as the "color of your transmission fluid", or you might think of it as flavor, wine flavor. Is it harsh and bitter, or is it gentle and light. Is it rough or smooth. Is it acidic or alkaline.

I just used the word, "rough". What do you think rough does inside the body? If you were to put rough wood-chips, or rough shattered-glass pieces into your bloodstream, what do you think would happen? They would scrape against the walls of the blood vessels and tear them up.

INFLAMMATION

Everyone is talking about inflammation as being the cause of many problems. This is true. Inflammation of the gums is gingivitis, gum disease. Inflammation of the arteries causes plaque buildup. Inflammation at the back of the eye, the retina, causes vision impairment.

So what causes inflammation? Well, there's inflammation that's caused by infection or injury, but the more common inflamers, are chemicals. We already talked about chlorine, but there's high blood sugar, free radicals, trans fat, food additives, air pollution, metals, plastics, medications, and on and on. But one cause of inflammation that I've never heard anyone mention is, acid. High-acidity low-alkalinity levels of the blood.

Recall that your blood pH range is 7.35 to 7.45. That's a very tight range. Five one-hundredths up from 7.4 and five one-hundredths down from 7.4. With a total range of $1/10^{th}$ of a whole number. What that tells me is, that pH is very critical to the body.

Recall that if your blood pH drops in alkalinity to that of plain water, i.e., from 7.4 to 7.0, you are circling-the-drain. And that if it drops to below 7.0 and stays there, just entering the acidic side, say, 6.9 and 6.8, you're dead.

So what do you think would happen if you had small pockets of low pH in your blood? Those pockets of acid would inflame the walls of the endothelial lining.

There are many things that cause inflammation. But by keeping your urine pH at exactly pH 7, and not at 6, and definitely not at 5, you can, in my opinion, cross off one inflammatory factor from your list.

CHAPTER 29

FACTS

This chapter will cite some textbook facts to help you understand the importance of keeping your urine at a neutral pH of 7.

From the book, *A Handbook of Routine Urinalysis* by Sister Laurine Graff, we find the following.

1. "One of the functions of the kidney is to help maintain acid-base balance in the body."

Whenever you see the word "base", just substitute "alkalinity", they are synonymous, and alkalinity just makes more sense. You wouldn't say, "I eat a base diet" but rather, "I eat an alkaline diet, high in fruits and vegetables and low in animal protein."

Do you find it interesting that there is so much public knowledge and talk about the heart, cancer, diabetes, lungs, thyroid, liver, pancreas, kidneys, gastrointestinal tract, gall bladder, brain, blood vessels, but no talk whatsoever about the INTERNAL STATE of the body? Acid-base balance is sort of like body temperature, which we know needs to be 98.6 degrees for optimum health, so too, the body has an optimum acid alkaline range, but it's virtually unheard of in the mainstream and healthcare. Why is that?

2. "To maintain a constant pH in the blood, the kidney must vary the pH of the urine to compensate for diet and products of

metabolism."

Products of metabolism produce either an alkaline ash, which occurs after you eat fruits and vegetables; or an acid ash, which occurs after you eat meat, fish, poultry, pork, eggs, and refined starches; or a neutral ash, from eating pretty much everything else. Foods that create a "slight" alkaline ash or "slight" acid ash, are not significant acid-base players. So, what this quote in this textbook is saying is, that the kidneys will change the pH of your urine to compensate for your diet. Therefore, if your urine is always acidic, your diet has excess acid byproducts. This is key.

Conversely, if your urine is always alkaline, then your diet has an excess of alkaline forming foods, which is rare in today's culture. Only a healthy vegan might see his or her urine pH above 7, exactly 7 yes, but not likely above 7.

I chose to target my urine pH at exactly 7 because 7 is neutral, it's not acidic, from excess acid, and it's not alkaline, from excess alkalinity. And we know that the pH of water is 7, and water is very neutral and soothing. It's also known that the pH of a cola drink is 4, acidic, and this is why people drink colas with their big high-calorie combo meals, to help provide additional acid for digestion. I was guilty of this. This is why the NCD meals are set to 500 calories. Not only does it make calorie counting simple and easy, but you avoid LARGE meals that make a person turn to colas, coffee, or sweets to give them a lift after eating.

Vinegar's another food that's an acid. Drink a tablespoon of apple cider vinegar on an empty stomach and you can feel the burning sensation. Plain white vinegar is much like the refined white flour refined white sugar and refined white salt, it's devoid. The ACV does contain the beneficial plant minerals from the apples, but it's still an acid. I have personally tried ACV as there are claims that it lowers blood pressure. Come to find out, it doesn't work for most people, and the reason stated is, that you have to alkalize the ACV with baking soda to get it to work. There's that baking soda thing again. It just keeps coming up no matter where you look. Anyway,

I don't take ACV as a supplement, I just use it in recipes, like in the NCD Chicken Caesar Salad™ dressing.

So by keeping your urine pH at exactly 7, you basically have neutral water exiting your kidneys.

There really isn't an alkaline problem going on in people's bodies today, it's an excess acid problem. There are four situations where the urine will appear alkaline, and they are, one, you have a UTI and the organism is *Proteus*, two, your alkaline reserves are used up and your body has switched to making ammonia to neutralize acid, three, your kidneys are damaged and they can't excrete acid into the urine, and four, you consumed too much bicarbonate. The first three conditions are pathological disease states, and these people need professional medical attention. The fourth condition occurs when you don't know your urine-pH numbers.

By keeping your urine pH at exactly 7, with the help of ABC Water, you are artificially creating in your body the environment of a young healthy vegetarian.™

3. "An alkaline urine can be induced with sodium bicarbonate, potassium citrate, and acetazolamide."

Or, as in the case of the highly-perfected formula of the ABC Water™, a combination of sodium and potassium bicarbonate.

In the textbook, *Urinalysis And Body Fluids* by Susan King Strasinger, the following statements can be found.

1. "To maintain a normal blood pH of 7.4 it is necessary to buffer and to eliminate the excess acid formed by dietary intake and body metabolism."

Again, the body is producing acid, that's what it does. The problem occurs when the body's "buffering" systems are running on empty. The body looks for alkalinity to maintain the blood pH at 7.4, but it can't find any.

2.   "The buffering capacity of the blood is dependent on bicarbonate ions, which are readily filtered by the glomerulus and must be expediently returned to the blood to maintain the proper pH."

This is key.   Your body is going to do everything possible to maintain your blood pH at 7.4.   So, you go to the doctor, he or she orders a Basic Metabolic Chemistry Panel, your Bicarbonate is in the normal range, and your doctor says, "You don't have an acidosis problem." Wrong. I just said, the blood is always going to have normal levels.   The deficiency is happening INSIDE THE CELLS and IN THE TISSUES. This is where the medical system and lab tests will misguide you into thinking you are okay when you're not. And you sense that you're not okay. That's why you went to the doctor.   Lab tests, aka, blood work, tests the blood only. Your body's number-one priority is the blood level. So, your body will take bicarbonate from other places. The same is true for iron, magnesium, calcium, and other nutrients as well. The body takes magnesium from the tissues to maintain blood levels.   The body takes calcium from the bones to maintain blood levels.   The body takes storage iron, ferritin, from the bone marrow to make iron for the blood.

Your blood levels are always going to be normal as long as you have supplies elsewhere to pull from.™

By the time the blood levels are abnormal, your body's supplies are depleted. The shelves in your pantry are empty. This is key.

When the doctor sends you to the lab for tests, the phlebotomist takes samples of your blood, not samples of your storage areas.

I believe aging is mostly caused by a person's body becoming depleted in one or more nutrients. By the time your depletion shows up in the blood, you have a problem that's already rooted. A problem that began years ago from something good that you weren't doing, or from something bad that you were doing, or a little of both.

3. "There are no normal values assigned to urinary pH, and it must be considered in conjunction with other patient information, such as the acid-base balance of the blood, the patient's renal function, the presence of urinary tract infection, and the patient's dietary intake, and the age of the specimen."

This is all true, but too lengthy to discuss fully here. I am cutting through the maze of details to give the reader the key points, the wisdom, and to make it understandable. The point here is, that if your doctor or anyone else says that the urine is supposed to be acidic, wrong, as "there are no normal values for urinary pH", as stated in this, and the other, urinalysis textbooks.

"The pH has to be considered in conjunction with the acid-base balance of the blood." Meaning, if your blood needs alkalinity, bicarbonate, it will take it from the urine and the urine will exit out the body as acidic, pH 5 or 6. This is an example of the body prioritizing the blood levels and taking supplies from elsewhere. Now, what about if the urine is low in alkalinity? What will happen? Where does the body go next? To the tissues. Your pantry.

Any time you see a urine pH of 5, that means your body is going to the pantry for supplies. When your pantry, cells and tissues, get low, because the blood has been stealing supplies from them, then things start to not work right. And this "not working right" can show up anywhere from the top of your head to the tip of your toe. That paragraph alone is worth the price of this book. Read it again.

Next. "The pH has to be considered in conjunction with the patient's renal function." If you have kidney damage, possibly from too much dietary protein and too much acid and not enough alkaline, your kidneys may not be able to excrete acid as much as they should, so your urine pH may appear as a 6 instead of a 5. This is similar to the smoker who holds on to carbon dioxide because his or her lungs are damaged and they can't exhale or blow off the bad stuff. As with the smoker retaining CO_2, the kidney-damaged person is retaining acid.

"The pH has to be considered in conjunction with the presence of a urinary tract infection." We've already discussed this. Certain bacteria can convert urea into ammonia, then, this ammonia neutralizes the acid in the urine to create an alkaline pH. This is not true alkalosis, this is, alkalosis due to bad bacteria, a UTI. The pH range in which the kidneys can make urine is 4.5 at the low end, and 8 at the upper end. So if you see a 9, which is typical of *Proteus*, and you have pain, cloudy and smell, see a doctor.

God gave us a natural solution for this problem. I find this so fascinating. Fruit and vegetable metabolism results in an alkaline ash, like the ash that remains after you burn a log in your fireplace. Cranberries are the exception to the rule. They produce an acid ash, so cranberries are over in the category with the meats and proteins. By drinking cranberry juice, fresh cranberries juiced in a blender with no sugar, you acidify the urine and flush out the *Proteus*. Cranberry juice also works to eliminate urinary tract infections caused by *Escherichia coli*, the bug responsible for 90% of all UTIs, but its effect is not pH related. Instead, the high mannose sugar content in cranberries coats the *E. coli* germ and prevents it from binding to the walls of the urinary tract. Isn't it amazing that this one berry was created as the oddball for this specific purpose? For you teenagers and young people out there that feel like you don't fit in, no worries, God has a specific purpose for you as well. You're the Cranberry! Go find your purpose.

"The pH has to be considered in conjunction with the patient's dietary intake." Here's the value. Here's the key. An acidic urine indicates that there wasn't enough bicarbonate base available so that the urine could leave the kidneys at a neutral pH of 7. Alkaline Shortage. And how does this happen? Diet.

This textbook only looks at diet and protein metabolism as a source of acid, but you know that there are two others, right? Exercise and Anxiety.

And the last one, "The pH has to be considered in conjunction with the age of the specimen." Meaning that the pH changes as it sits around exposed to air, so test immediately.

In summary, there are no normal values for urinary pH, as stated in the textbooks, so if anyone says the pH of the urine is supposed to be acidic, ask them to show you where it says that in the textbooks. It may say that urine pH is USUALLY or OFTEN acidic, but that's different than NORMAL.

A urine pH of 5 is telling you about your internal alkaline reserves.

CHAPTER 30

Prescription Medication

So you ask, is this okay to do if I am taking XYZ medication for XYZ problem? The answer is clear, NO.

If you are taking prescription medication, you are by definition under the care of your physician. This book is for the Selfcare Individual, the person who's under their own care.

Any medical professional will tell you that you can't take prescription medication and then try to do your own thing on the side. It just doesn't work that way. Medications are serious. Iatrogenic death, deaths that result from medical treatment, is the third leading cause of death in the United States. Read Dr. Ray Strand's book, *Death By Prescription*. Funny, we never hear about the number three cause of death. We only hear that cancer and heart disease are number one and two. Sometimes they will say that lung disease is number four, but we never hear about number three. Hm. Is somebody trying to hide something? Ask anyone what the third leading cause of death is and they won't know. They also will have never heard the word "iatrogenic" before. If you worry about heart disease and cholesterol or getting cancer, then you should likewise worry about dying as a result of prescription medication.

The point is, you either control your own care and take responsibility for your own state of health, or lack thereof, OR, you are under the control of your physician and are following his plan for your care and health, or lack thereof. But you can't do both. It's dangerous. And tens of thousands of people die every year from adverse reactions while taking prescription drugs.

This book never mentions how prescription drugs affect urine pH because prescription drugs are incompatible with a selfcare guide. If you are taking prescription drugs this book is not for you. You are under the control and responsibility of your physician and you don't deviate from his instructions and try to do your own thing.

You are free to read this book for informational purposes only. And, you are free to decide who you want controlling your health, and what your future holds.

For those of you who want to get off of your prescription medications for whatever reasons you may have, I recommend following the advice of Dr. Lorraine Day, whose credits include that of being an ER trauma surgeon, as well as being a, to-the-grave-and-back cancer survivor, and now she's 74 years old and looking literally half her age.

I wouldn't concern yourself with double-blind studies regarding this that or the other, but rather, just study what Dr. Day recommends and do that. That's my advice. Her website again is, www.drday.com.

CHAPTER 31

CONSPIRACY

Yes, I'm going there. Why do people think conspiracies don't happen? On the contrary, they are happening all around us, and have been throughout history. Two or more people meeting in private to change the direction of things. An agenda is a conspiracy that's out in the open. But conspiracy implies a bit more, a covering up, a hiding of the truth, by either lying, or omission of key facts.

As the main character in the New Testament once said, which still applies today, "And ye shall know the truth, and the truth shall make you free." John 8.32

Knowing the truth should empower you, so that as changes are occurring, you find yourself equipped with the tools you need to navigate your way through the game of life, making it around the board, passing obstacles, to the end, home free, unscathed. "Yay! I won!"

Looking back on my life, those "Tools" have been Information.

INFORMATION PRODUCTS

I've spent hundreds of dollars on information products and don't regret one penny of it. I got my first set of Brian Tracy tapes at the age of 15 and began setting clear written-down goals, and keeping my thoughts focused on those goals, like a homing device.

Interestingly though, goal setting is about you homing in on what you want, but what's cool about goal setting is, WHAT YOU WANT WANTS YOU. So as you move towards your goal, your goal moves towards you. This is the Divine Hand of the Universe at work, conspiring on your behalf. Every few steps you take towards your goal, through work, effort, reading, productivity, the Divine Hand also moves that goal a few steps in your direction.

School books are one kind of information, the information that everybody learns, aka, common knowledge. Information Products are a completely different kind of information, uncommon knowledge. Information Products are for a few select group of people, for the elite, traditionally, but now everyone has access to them. You can put yourself in that group of elite by simply reading what they read and knowing what they know. The price of this book is a reflection of its value, in that, you could potentially save yourself thousands if not tens-of-thousands of dollars in medical bills by steering yourself away from a heart bypass, cancer treatment, a kidney transplant, and dozens of others, by following what I have outlined in this book.

The leaders of society, the CEOs CFOs, business owners, politicians, doctors, lawyers, are all people who seek inside information, whether it be in the area of health, finance, economics, sales, relationships, what-have-you. If you are a parent, I encourage you to add Information Products to your children's education, if you want to raise them up from the masses and the competition. Much like how information about a particular company can give you an advantage in the stock market and make you wealthy, so too can information, "Insider Information", about health, wellness, and disease, give you an advantage as you journey your way through life.

So my story begins with a television program I watched today, where one doctor was interviewing another doctor, a nephrologist, kidney doctor. Now, let me start by saying that these two men are very fine professionals who do a tremendous amount of good. BUT, there are some key words they just would not say or discuss. The interview was one-hour long and the words "pH" "acid" "acidosis" "alkaline" "alkalosis" "bicarbonate" and "acid-base balance" were never used.

Now the kidney's primary role is to filter blood. Once job number one is done, its second job is to, REABSORB BICARBONATE IONS BACK IN TO THE KIDNEY SO THAT THIS PRECIOUS ALKALIZING SUBSTANCE CAN BE USED TO MAINTAIN THE BLOOD PH AT 7.4, AKA, ACID-BASE BALANCE.

Now, both doctors know this. Nurses and Medical Lab Scientists know this. That the function of the kidney is to filter the blood, and to reabsorb bicarbonate, and excrete excess acid, in order to maintain acid-base balance in the blood.

What they did discuss were, the progressive steps towards end-stage kidney disease, other health conditions that can lead to kidney disease, lab tests that diagnose kidney disease, treatment options for kidney patients, and supplements to support health if you have already been diagnosed with kidney damage.

I kept waiting for this highly-regarded nephrologist to say something like, you've got to get these people on a high-alkaline diet of fruits and vegetables and cut back on dietary protein to correct the excess-acid problem. Well, at one point he did mention the vegetarian diet, but he referred to it as a "Phytochemical Diet". Phytochemical, or phytonutrient, just means color pigments, which is true, plants contain the most color nutrients. But a vegetarian diet is an alkaline diet, and it's the alkalinity which is the reason why sick people often turn to juicing fruits and vegetables as a way to improve their condition. Both doctors refused to use the word "alkaline" "alkalinity" or "base". Conspiracy Fact #1

At one point the nephrologist was giving an example of a patient who had ended-up in the ER and was diagnosed with kidney disease, and finally he said this, "They have diminished reserves."

But he jumbled his words and mumbled as he said it. My question to you mister nephrologist is, Diminished Reserves of WHAT?

Then he went on to say that the condition could be caused by pneumonia, viral infections, nausea, vomiting, and diarrhea. One of the kidney's primary jobs is ACID MANAGEMENT. But no mention of acid, or acidosis. Conspiracy Fact #2. In fact, "vomiting" is outright misinformation, because vomiting removes stomach acid from the body, resulting in an alkaline state.

Sadly, the average viewer of this program would not have caught all of the, what I will call as, mild-to-moderate deception for the sole purpose of winding up the program with a long list of supplements. Shame shame. But this is the free market. You snooze you lose. And the uninformed, or misinformed, pay dearly for their lack of knowledge. Hosea 4.6 says they are "destroyed".

I've watched this program before and they've had other guests on, one is a notable cardiologist, who, admitted on TV that he used to recommend margarine to his patients. That's criminal in my opinion. Trans fat is worse than rancid fat. When they asked scientists what would be the allowable limit that could be put on the Nutrition Facts label, the scientists said, NONE, trans fat is toxic, having the same effects as poison.

You would be wise to look closely at the details of the people you are following for advice. Who's behind it, man or God?

Another thing that I've noticed upon viewing their programs, is that they try to talk over people's heads to make themselves appear as informed cutting-edge experts who want to help the viewer get well. In doing so, they talk quickly, they cut off a sentence at the end and never finish it, throw in things that sound fancy but aren't related or relevant, and basically create a PERFORMANCE or a SHOW. My heart goes out to the millions of viewers who work as engineers, truck drivers, clerks, social workers, and don't have a good grasp of biochemistry, science, physiology, and medical terminology, who are looking for clear concise steps, but instead end up with just haphazardly buying and taking this or that supplement.

Conspiracy Fact #3
Later on, the nephrologist said, "Something is putting them over the edge." He knows darn-well what that "Something" is but wouldn't say it. Shame shame. I just wrote an entire book about that "Something", empowering the reader with a complete guide to take control of that "Something". But they just wouldn't say the word. Acidosis.

This next one isn't a conspiracy, but more like a backwards way of looking at a problem. Picture a garden hose attached to a water tap, and on the other end is a spray nozzle. Now, turn the tap half-a-turn. What happens? Well, water fills the hose. What else is happening? Well, the hose, which was flat, is now filled up and round, there is pressure being exerted on the inside wall of the hose. And there is pressure in the nozzle. Okay. Now turn the tap all-the-way open, creating maximum water pressure in the hose. Now, go over to the nozzle, squeeze the trigger, and flip up the metal piece to lock the trigger in the open position, and adjust the screw on the trigger so that the water leaving is at maximum, 100%, a fully-squeezed trigger. This is your kidney.

The pressure in the hose, tube, vessel, is normal, firm but soft. There is 100% flow or filtration of the liquid, water, or blood, entering the spray-nozzle kidney.

Now, what would happen if sand, particles, and debris, came through your tap and entered the hose? Well, it would travel down the hose vessel and when it reached the intricate interior structure of the spray-nozzle kidney, it would begin to clog it up. Some of the sand, particles, and debris would leave, but some of it would not. This condition continues, and you notice that one hour later, you only have 75% of the water coming out of the nozzle. What is happening to the walls of the garden hose? Well, that backed-up water is creating more pressure on the walls. Two hours later, you notice that you have even less water coming out of the spray nozzle, about half or 50%. You also notice that your garden hose is very solid and pumped up.

When the sand, particles, and debris have clogged up your spray nozzle to the extent that you have only 15% of the water leaving the spray nozzle, you are on dialysis and are looking at getting a kidney transplant.

But what about the garden hose? What is happening to the walls of the garden hose? Well, they started out as firm but soft, and now they are tight, pumped, and under a lot of pressure. This is your blood pressure.

So, I ask you this. Did the pressure cause the kidneys to fail? No. The kidney damage caused the pressure to increase.

It's the, "Which came first the chicken or the egg?" situation again. The medical mindset says, including these two doctors on TV, that "High Blood Pressure Causes Kidney Damage." Really. So what causes high blood pressure? Well, doctors don't know, that's why it's called essential hypertension, we don't know what causes it.

The premise is backwards, the medical mindset is blaming the "chicken".

The kidney, spray nozzle, gets damaged, and then the blood pressure goes up, in the garden hose. It's not the pressure in the garden hose that damages the kidneys, because in the beginning, before the sand and debris clogged the spray nozzle, the pressure in the garden hose was normal, firm but soft.

Now, once the kidneys get damaged, and the blood pressure goes up, then the system feeds back on itself and the two problems compound together, the more the kidneys get damaged the higher the blood pressure, and the higher the blood pressure the more damage to the kidneys, so you're in a vicious cycle and a downward spiral, unless you can get the sand out of the spray nozzle and get the water 100% flowing again.

I can't help but think that these two doctors know this, but are misinforming the public on purpose to maintain their profession and livelihood. Oh, you say "doctors wouldn't do that". Oh really. Ask a chiropractor to what extent the medical profession will go to protect their business interests.

Now in their defense, this TV program has come out and stated that high cholesterol has very little to do with heart disease and that statin drugs are not effective in most patients, and that statin drugs actually CAUSE heart disease by blocking the pathway that produces co-enzyme Q10, CoQ10.   This is very noble of them. Telling the truth and going against your profession and colleagues takes a lot of bravery and you put yourself at risk by doing so. This program has also given dozens of other good and valuable pieces of advice, and I personally purchase some of the products they promote.

BUT.   This particular program was clearly a sales pitch to sell supplements and the way it was done was shameful.

Hence my belief that acidosis, excess acid, your internal fluid color, and its opposite, alkalosis, fruits and vegetables, bicarbonate, are key underlying components to a healthy body, and that, if you kept them in balance, might potentially jeopardize an entire industry, so shhh, quiet.

CHAPTER 32

The Medical System

I want to be clear that I am not bashing the medical system. It's doing what it has been set up to do. And it does that well, and very well in some areas. If you go to the hospital with a problem, they use all the tools at their disposal to find and diagnose the problem and then treat it. Many many lives have been saved.

The part of the medical system that I don't care for is its lack of addressing the root of the problem, and so people continue down a rabbit hole of treatment-upon-treatment, hoping to someday get better. But the medical system does exactly what it's set up to do. It is up to the individual to learn a little bit about health and disease and take an active role in getting better.

This is where self-help books and books written by people who have gone through the same thing can be life changing. It is the patient's job to find the answer, not the medical system's. It can be compared to the school system. If you don't like the education your kids are getting, you are free to do-it-yourself, homeschool them, or with regard to healthcare, you are free to do selfcare.

The medical system is not there to find the answer to your problem, it's there to do what it's set up to do, diagnose, test, monitor, and treat disease according to their model.

If you want answers it's up to you to go out and find them. It is not the medical system's job to give you the answers, tell you the complete truth, or fix your problem. Their only job is to execute protocols set up by the system. So, there is no fault whatsoever in the medical system. They are doing exactly what they are outlined to do.

It's the patient's fault for believing that the medical system is the cure for their problem, and for thinking that the medical system is going to make everything in their body function right. It doesn't work that way. The medical system treats problems based on established protocols. For every patient out there that claims that the medical system failed them, I say, wrong. You failed you.

You are responsible for finding the answers to your health ailments. You are responsible for recognizing when you are making choices on autopilot instead of thinking about what you are really eating and drinking, putting on your skin, cleaning with, and all of the other lifestyle habits you expose yourself to. You can not blame the medical system, and I surely do not. It's their system and it's set up their way. That's their right to do so.

Now if it was me, I would set it up a little differently, with a lot more education, a lot more personal responsibility, and a lot more root cause treatments.

If you enter the medical system for treatment for a problem and they save you and get you back on your feet again, Fantastic! They are pros at this in many ways. But if you feel yourself spiraling downward year-by-year and you are getting frustrated with your medical treatment, that's your fault. There are hundreds of alternatives out there, thousands of personal testimonies, and many many people who have found the root cause to the exact same problem you have. You just have to look.

You have to take personal responsibility for handing the reins of your care over to a system that tells you up front that, they can "do this or that but there's no guarantee". They may or may not know the underlying cause of your condition, but if they do, they don't have to tell you.

I took my dress shoes to the cobbler and had them polished. When I picked them up they looked brand new. I asked him, "How did you make these shoes look brand new?" The shoeshiner said, "It's a secret." Do you think your Financial Advisor is going to tell you all he knows? Of course not. So don't expect the medical system to tell you their secret knowledge either.

If you don't know the secrets to investing or polishing your shoes, or health or medical, it's your own fault. When you fail to take PERSONAL RESPONSIBILITY in any area of your life, and it goes badly, you are the one to blame.

I've recommended professional medical treatment several times in this book because I know, and everyone knows, that certain conditions require medical treatment.

But the fact that they never talk about your Internal Environment, or they say diet isn't the cause, or they say cancer and high blood pressure just happen, that's their prerogative. They can tell you full truths, half truths, or no truths, it's their system. You have to SEEK the truth yourself to find the answers to your problem.

If you're going to make it through the game of life and come out on the other side a winner, like Dr. Lorraine Day, you had better do your research. And take Personal Responsibility. "If it's to be, it's up to me", Brian Tracy.

CHAPTER 33

Add-ons

There's another thing I would like to mention regarding anyone who says that your urine pH is supposed to be acidic and that 5 and 6 are normal, when they aren't normal, they are merely common. The fact is, that if the doctor's clients were all vegetarians, then a urine pH of 7 would be common.

But here's an interesting fact. White vinegar has a pH of 4.5, that's what's written in the literature and I tested mine and sure enough the color is halfway between 4 and 5 using the 0-13 paper, and using my other pH paper it was 4.5 exactly. So, if your urine pH is 5, according to your urinalysis result from your lab workup, then you are only one-half a step away from having urine that's like white vinegar. Imagine bathing your poor hard-working kidneys in white vinegar 24 hours a day, or even 2 hours a day, or even 10 minutes. No thank you.

Also, laboratory dipstick tests for urine pH only go as low as pH 5. However, your kidneys can actually create urine with a pH of 4.5. So, if your urinalysis result says pH 5, it could be 5 or 4.5, you don't know, because the lower limit of the pH dipstick test is 5.

I have thought about this while working on the bench in the urinalysis department. Laboratories should really be reporting the result as less-than or equal to five, ≤ 5. Because it could be 5 or it could be 4.5. You don't know. If the machine says 5, it gets reported as 5, but it could be 4.5.

The reason an additional one-half a whole number is significant, is because pH is a logarithmic scale. Meaning, that every step is times ten. So a half a step, is times five. Therefore, a urine pH of 4.5 is five-times more acidic than a urine pH of 5. To me, this is significant.

Think back to our car driving on the freeway at 70 mph, as a way of looking at keeping our urine pH at exactly 7, and we locked in the cruise-control button. When our urine pH drops from 7 to 6, our speed actually drops from 70 mph to 7 mph. Because each step on the pH scale is times ten. Now if we continue in an acid state, eating meat and insufficient fruits and vegetables, exercising, negative thinking, then our pH drops from 6 to 5, our car speed now drops from 7 mph, to 0.7 mph, or 7/10ths of a mile per hour.

If you run on a treadmill, you know that 7 mph is a good challenging run speed. You're running but not sprinting. Now picture a funeral setting, and people walking away from the site, they are walking very slowly, this is about 0.7 miles per hour.

So think of a urine pH of 5 as being the walk speed of those at a funeral, and think of a urine pH of 6 as running, almost sprinting, on a treadmill, then think of driving on the freeway at 70 miles per hour as the urine pH of 7.

And then you wonder why I avoid 5 like the plague, and if I drop into the sixes, I quickly take corrective action, 3-4 sips of ABC Water™.

In my opinion, your urine pH is your speed, energy, and performance. You can be Zoom Zoom, or you can be dragging your feet. Or you can do what so many people do. And that is, they're dragging, so they stimulate their body with caffeine and voila, Zoom Zoom again!

This is a very dangerous long-term situation, because you are using caffeine, a performance-enhancing drug, according to the Olympic Rules, just ask that female gymnast who was disqualified when caffeine showed up in her urine from drinking a diet coke.

Don't cheat. It's not an honest way to live your life. This includes stimulants, of any kind.   The Number Crunch Diet™ has a No Caffeine Rule. Your goal is to figure out a way to make your body have its own energy. Not drug it into performing for you.

Caffeine masks the underlying condition.   That of acidosis. Fatigue.

So if you continue this pattern of using caffeine to keep you going, your body becomes progressively more acidic, until, one day, crash, you end up in the hospital.

But what if you could raise your zoom zoom by raising your alkaline status?

Going back to our urine that could actually be pH 4.5, and you can see it for yourself by using your 0-13 paper and if the color is halfway between 4 and 5 you can say it's 4.5, the "speed" of this urine pH is 0.3 miles per hour. This would be equivalent to the speed of a baby crawling across the living room floor.

I will bet money on this next statement being true.   The people with urine pHs of 5 or 4.5 are using caffeine on a daily basis to stimulate their bodies to perform.

Now, let's go back to our acetic-acid white vinegar with its pH of 4.5. On an empty stomach, swallow one ounce of white vinegar. I suggest you have a glass of water nearby because it's going to burn. Now a urine with a pH of 4.5 is the same thing. And 5 is not far behind.   Another protein meal, exercise class, or a hateful emotion, and your funeral walk 5 drops down to a baby crawl 4.5.

Could kidney damage, damage to the filtering nets of the kidneys, be due to the "nets" being curdled from soaking in vinegar?

Isn't "pickling" when you soak something in vinegar?

If vinegar, in the absence of food, burns the walls of your stomach lining, causing irritation, inflammation, and repeated offenses leading to stomach ulcers and blood in the stool, why would you do this same thing to your kidneys?

Wisdom is the principle key. Saying that your urine should be acidic, is like the cardiologist in the 1980s telling his patients to use margarine. Or the family doctor who tells his overweight patient to go on a low-fat diet, which can only mean one thing, you consume more carbs. And then the patient comes back on her next visit having gained 3-5 pounds.

I am going to take a moment to applaud you for reading this book up to this point. I believe I have thrown a lot of material at you and you stuck with it. You my friend, have the makings of a winner, a person with wisdom, who will navigate herself or himself through life with a keen eye.

If what I have written makes sense to you, maybe you already knew of the importance of alkalinity but just weren't sure how to implement supplementation, or you didn't know how to determine your current acid alkaline status, then recommend my book to a friend, or coworker, a family member. Basically, anyone you know of that's drinking caffeine for energy would benefit by switching to ABC Water™.   But have them read the book, so that they understand fully what it's all about. Thank you for your support.

To close this chapter, let's look at our logarithmic pH scale again. So you know that half a step is times five, and a full step is times ten. This means that, when you go from pH 7 to pH 6 you drop down by times ten, "70mph to 7mph". But, also realize that, pH 7 to pH 5 is times one hundred, "70mph to 0.7mph". That's a big drop. A urine pH of 5 is very acidic. That's my point. But what's more acidic is the 4.5 urine pH. This is 500 times more acidic than pH 7, 10x10x5=500. Wow. And people wonder why they're tired.

CHAPTER 34

Fruit Test Sunday™

Some of you may be familiar with other ways of testing your pH, such as saliva, the lemon juice test, the protein challenge, these are fine but I came up with my own. I like it and it's safe and simple.

Pick one day, Sunday would be a good day, where you will eat nothing but fruit the entire day. Previously I referred to this as Fat Free Sunday™, where I also eat fat-free chicken breast coated with BBQ sauce. For this Fruit Test Sunday™, you will omit the protein, as well as the fat, and eat only fruit.

Prepare for this day by purchasing a 5 lb bag of valencia oranges, 2 lbs of grapes, and a watermelon.

Prep it in advance the day before by washing the grapes and removing the stems, discarding any soft grapes, and dividing them into two bowls. The large pyrex bowls with the red lids at Walmart work good. So your 2 lbs of grapes becomes two servings of about 14oz of grapes, which is about 250 calories per serving, 500 calories for both.

Wash the outside of your watermelon with hot water, towel dry it, and place it on the kitchen counter. Using a long bread knife, the one with a serrated blade, like a steak knife, cut the ends off the watermelon, like how you would cut the ends off a lemon. Now, turn the watermelon 90 degrees to sit it on its end. Cut the peel off

137

in strips, in downward slices, until you have removed all the peel. You can flip it over to sit it on its other end if you need to. Discard the peel. Cut the watermelon in half lengthwise, and place the two halves face down on your counter. Next, cut through the middle of each half watermelon, creating a double layer. Now, slice and dice, slice lengthwise and then slice widthwise. Congratulations! You just prepared a 25-pound watermelon into bite-sized chunks. But you're not done yet. You need to get your watermelon into containers. The word for this is "Aliquoting".

An aliquot is a portion of the whole, similar to a serving, BUT, a measured serving, a calculated serving. This is different than a slice of cake or a spoonful of sour cream. An aliquot of food is a calculated, number crunched, serving. This word usage is Unique to the Number Crunch Diet. Aliquot – the new term in dieting.™

So, in the case of our watermelon, we are going to aliquot it, divide it, into 30oz servings using our large pyrex bowls with the red lids.

Place the bowl on your kitchen scale and press "tare" to zero it. Now, add 30 ounces of watermelon. Press on the lid and refrigerate it. Continue doing this until all of the watermelon is aliquoted into bowls. If you have a few pieces left over, just add them to some of your servings (1oz more is only 8 calories, no biggie) or reward yourself with a little fresh watermelon. Mmm!

When you are done you may have anywhere from 8 to 12 servings of watermelon, depending on the size of your watermelon and how thinly you cut the peel off.

Each of these 30oz servings of watermelon is about 250 calories.

By now I hope you understand the importance of your kitchen tools. The glass pyrex bowls for storing food you prepare, the scale, the bread knife, etc.

I purchased my kitchen scale at Smart & Final grocery and restaurant-supply store. My prior scale was purchased at Walmart, but the maximum capacity was 5 lbs. The S&F scale goes up to 10 lbs and later on you will see that this comes in handy when dividing up big batches of food, as you will want to know the total weight of the batch before you divide it up.

It's made by Taylor, the TE10C digital scale with power cord, and it cost $50. Don't buy one that runs on batteries. Also, don't buy one that shuts off quickly. This TE10C stays on until I decide to shut it off.

The bread knife is made by Sani-Safe, also available at S&F, for about $13. The blade is 12-inches long, making it perfect for cutting up melons, as well as for making breadsticks, as I will explain in the NCD Sausage Pizza™ recipe. This bread knife, and the 10-inch cutting knife, S&F Chef's Review $12, are the only two knives I use to prepare 90% of my food.

A restaurant-supply store like S&F is a great place to shop for big job items, like the bigger scale capacity, the bigger bread knife, big cans of pumpkin, big cans of sauerkraut, ginormous cans of tuna. Just be sure to read the label because some of the products have undesirable ingredients. The big can of tomato paste has one ingredient, tomatoes. It doesn't get much simpler than that.

So now you're prepped and ready for your Fruit Test Sunday™.

Now, a word of caution, if you are diabetic, you are under the care of your doctor, so this is not something you would do, or anyone with blood-sugar regulatory problems.

Your FTS might look like this.
07:00 Up
07:30 4 valencia oranges, about 250 calories
10:00 4 valencia oranges
12:30 14oz of grapes, bowl #1
15:00 14oz of grapes, bowl #2
17:30 30oz of watermelon
20:00 30oz of watermelon

23:00 lights out

Okay. Your day is over and you've had six servings of fruit, each being 250 cals, so your total caloric intake was 1500 calories. This is a low calorie day, but all of your calories came from sugar, so you don't want to go too high for your daily total calories. Additionally, those 250cal fruit meals were spaced 2.5 hours apart. Most people will burn 100 calories an hour just doing normal activities, so 2.5 hours times 100 calories is 250 calories. You shouldn't gain weight using this One-hundred-Calories-per-Hour™ rule. Also notice that the last meal was 3 hours before bed, so your last serving of watermelon should be burned off before you turn out the lights, and thus, you shouldn't be storing sugar as fat while you sleep nor having dumb dreams because your brain is awake.

When I do a Fat Free Sunday, I have 250cals of fruit every two hours, that's eight servings, totaling 2000 calories. Plus I have two servings of lean chicken breast. If you boil trimmed lean chicken breast in water, all of the fat leaves the chicken and it becomes NCD Fat Free Chicken™. Slice and dice the chicken breast, aliquot it into your 8oz glass jars that you purchased at SKS, add some BBQ sauce, cap and shake, and voila, BBQ chicken with no fat. Deeelicious!

So my FFS consists of 2000 calories of fruit, 400 calories of fat-free protein, and 100 calories of the sauce, totaling 2500 calories for the day. I don't gain weight doing this. For you workout enthusiasts, this is a great way to carb-load your muscles for your next week of workouts. You wake up Monday morning charged, stocked, and ready-to-go!

I am sure you have heard of this popular concept called the "Cheat Day". The NCD does not buy into this. Yes, you need to reset your metabolism and shock your body out of its normal eating habits every so often, but you don't do it with ice cream. The "Cheat Day", the way most people are doing it, even the advisors, is a two step backwards day. One author of a book said he eats a half-gallon of ice cream on his cheat day, oh that's brilliant advice.

You can also reset leptin, your appetite and hunger hormone, and shock your metabolism back into gear by doing Sweat Cardio™.

This whole "Cheat Day" advice started with someone who once lost a lot of weight, becoming an "expert", but has since gained a lot of fat on his waist. So clearly, he's been cheating.

JPM advice is based on putting in effort to gain long-term real results. It's not about cheating.

There are some Sundays where I may not do the FFS, and I just stick with 40% carbs, 30% fat, and 30% protein meals. Other Sundays, I may do HFFS or Half-day Fat Free Sunday™. It all depends on how you feel. If you feel good, recovered, with plenty of motivation and energy, you don't need a carb-load day. If you're partially recovered and motivated with okay energy but not good energy, then do HFFS. If Friday you worked out hard, and now Saturday you feel like you've been hit by a bus, then carb-load on Sunday and do the full day FFS.

You don't just eat carbs mindlessly.™

Carbs are your fuel source. If you mindlessly eat carbs without checking to see if you really need them or not, then you overfill your tank and the excess turns to fat.

It is common-sense sentences like the one you have just read that separates the Number Crunch Diet™ from the others.

Carb are like money.™ You have to earn them. And you don't spend $20 bills, or eat carbs, that you haven't earned. Because if you do, you will end up in debt, or fat. Or both.

YOU HAVE TO EARN YOUR CARBS, LIKE YOU EARN MONEY. YOU DON'T JUST SPEND MONEY, OR EAT CARBS, YOU HAVEN'T EARNED.™

Now back to your FTS test results. You should have been taking your urine pH throughout the day and recording your results. With all that liquid fruit, oranges, grapes, and especially the watermelon, you should have had several urinations this day.

The urine should reflect the alkalinity in the fruit and result in a urine pH of 7. If by the end of the day, 21:00, after your last bowl of 30oz watermelon, if your urine pH did not hit 7, you are alkaline deficient or depleted.

If your urine pHs were mostly 6s on this day, I call this Deficient. Half a tank remaining.

If your urine pHs were mostly 5s on this day, I call this Depleted. An eighth of a tank remaining.

A Healthy person with sufficient alkaline reserves doesn't need to soak up all the alkalinity from the six meals of fruit. Hence, that fruit alkalinity is not needed for storage and it goes out the urine and shows up as a urine pH of 7. This is what you want. Your pantry shelves, your body's tissues, are stocked with alkalinity.

The Deficient person soaked up some of the excess alkalinity from the fruit and so only some of the fruit alkalinity went out the urine and he or she had urine pHs in the sixes.

The Depleted person soaked up all of the alkalinity from the fruit and their urine pHs never turned alkaline, their urine pHs were in the fives, 5, and 5.5.

If you picture a pantry with shelves for storing food, you have the deficient person with half the shelves full and half the shelves empty.

The depleted person's pantry would be 80-90% empty shelves.

This is just my way of expressing the concept to you so that you get it. Do not quote me on the percentages or on this being an exact formula. It's a guide. This entire book is a guide. Based on my personal observations and experimentation with alkalinity and urine pH.

The take-home message is, that if you eat nothing but oranges grapes and watermelon all day, by the middle of the day, or the end of the day at the latest, your urine pH should be 7. If at the end of the day you never hit 7, you're low on alkaline reserves.

CHAPTER 35

CONCLUSION

As we conclude this discussion of ABC Water™ and related aspects, I think some things are worth repeating.

Although the bulk of what you have just read pertained to acid-base balance and my belief that maintaining your urine pH at 7 will make you feel better, and quite possibly, limitless more benefits, the significance of providing your body with a steady supply of vitamin B for energy and stress reduction, and vitamin C for repair, rebuild, and rejuvenation, should not be overlooked.

The emphasis was on the "A" because you already know about the "B" and the "C". The problem is, no one is talking about the "A". Why won't anyone talk about your INTERNAL ENVIRONMENT when it's just as important as your heart, liver, lungs, or brain.

Nurses know this. Patient comes into the ER, mid 50s, chest pain, abdominal obesity, shortness of breath, Arterial Blood Gas results show that the patient's blood pH is 7.1, she gives the patient Bicarbonate.

And if you've been a nurse for a while, then you've also seen the following situation occur. The bicarbonate's given, you draw another ABG expecting that the patient's blood pH will be normal, and surprise! It's still 7.1. How come? We gave the bicarb, the pH is supposed to go up.

If you read this book from the beginning, and you didn't just skim over the material, but you really read it and understood it before moving on to the next paragraph, then you should know the answer to this situation. Why didn't the patient's pH go up after giving the Bicarbonate?

Tick Tock Tick Tock Tick Tock...time's up.

Because the tissues are alkaline depleted and when they gave the bicarbonate the body just soaked it up.

This is a terrible condition to be in. Not only are you dying, and your body's intelligence in an attempt to save you, runs to the pantry for supplies, and there's nothing there. The shelves have been wiped out. And now you're getting help from the outside, an IV infusion, and that's still not enough.

Luckily for this patient, the nurse is relentless and determined to save her patient's life and she just keeps giving bicarb in massive amounts until the ABG results show a normal pH of 7.4.

Now if this patient had maintained a urine pH of exactly 7, the story would be different. In fact, there would be no story at all.

But it's not just this patient that's at risk, the over-exerciser with a high protein low fruit and vegetable diet, that, on the surface seems like he's in great physical shape, but has an underlying acidosis problem. Signs of fatigue that perhaps he or she has been masking with caffeine, tylenol, or worse, steroids, to allow the athlete to continue to push themselves. An acidosis problem that the coach, trainer, or physician can't detect because blood tests don't tell you about your alkaline stores.   Lab tests check blood levels, not "pantry" levels.

And then there's the slow drip condition, where every day and every week, month by month, your transmission fluid becomes a little darker.   Then one day, you can't drive your car and the mechanic tells you you've fried your transmission. "How did I do that?" you ask. "Well, you never paid attention to the fluid."

Lastly, it's always a good idea to take a break every now and then for a week or so, and I do this. I divide my year into quarters, 13 weeks times 4 quarters, think of a deck of 52 cards being the 52 weeks of a year, and then 13 of each of the 4 suits. I review at the end of the quarter to see if I'm on track with my goals and make adjustments if needed, aka, a quarterly review.

On the 13th week of each quarter I completely abandon my routine and do as much opposite as I can. This creates contrast, and snaps you out of any monotony that can occur from repeating your weeks over and over. It's like a vacation, but with an emphasis on doing everything different from your normal routine.

So, I stop taking supplements and exercising and reading and no internet, no television, no radio, and I spend time getting close to the earth. Each day I will lie on my back on the grass and allow my body internals to realign with the earth. Stopping your busy life and lying on the earth is a great way to decompress and destress. Mother earth just refreshes and cleans away any of the junk energies that don't need to be there.

During this week, I also stop driving, but instead I walk or ride my bike to any of the places that I need to go. It's a bit like getting OFF THE GRID for a week. You unplug. Don't worry, the grid will still be there when your week is over. If you've ever watched the movie *The Matrix*, it shows that there are two worlds, the Grid or Matrix world, that's not really real, and then the sort of real reality world.

So, take a step back every so often and skip the ABC Water™. But do take your urine pH, this I continue to do, as I like to see what effect it has. By the third day my urines are 5s. But then I will get some 6s and maybe a 7, as I do have good alkaline stores now. As the Off-Grid week comes to an end, you will find your motivation and drive for success and achievement are pumped up again and you will be ready to plug back into the Matrix and go go go!

CHAPTER 36

the bashers

Before the internet, if someone didn't support or agree with what you wrote or said, they would post a review or talk about it on a TV program. This commentary was generally clean, as far as language was concerned. With the internet however, one can say anything they want and be as foul as they choose to be, and I call these people the bashers.

I once made a positive comment on YouTube in favor of a political candidate that wasn't the mainstream's choice. Within minutes, the bashers came out and just batted my comment and me personally into a pulp. Interesting.

It was as though these people are professionals at this. As though they do this for a living. That they are combing the internet, looking for anything that doesn't mesh with their AGENDA, and they bash, defame, and name call, to get you and your idea to disappear from the list of choices.

To these people that do this, and should they post bashing name-calling comments about this book or me personally, I ask, "Who Do You Work For?"

What group or organization is my book a threat to? So much so that they asked you to damage, defame, and name call it out of existence. By doing so, not only do you make yourself look foolish, you prove that this book can have a powerful effect on improving people's lives, with a potential loss of customers for a certain group or industry.

I recently saw a doctor on TV state that, they will never do studies on such-and-such because they don't want to find the answers, because finding the answers would negatively impact their livelihood and profession.

And so it is with alkalosis. The subject rarely discussed in the mainstream, and yet so important to good health, and its opposite, acidosis, playing a key role in so many ailments.

As a final comment to the skeptics and those that may still be a little unsure about keeping your urine pH at 7, then drop your target pH to 6.5, and use the ABC Water to keep your urine pH at 6.5. So to any skeptics, I say this, if your urine pH is always in the 5s, you are a ticking time bomb, healthwise. No one can argue with that.

Chapter Endnote

Selectivity. What gets into the mainstream is very controlled by people at the top. It's also controlled by companies with massive advertising budgets. Word-of-mouth marketing is still the most effective way to spread the word. If you believe that people should have self-health options available to them, then kindly assist in using your voice or social platform to get the word out. Thank you, and may a fourfold blessing return your way.

CHAPTER 37

the NUMBER CRUNCH DIET ™

Okay, we are going to switch gears to the diet plan portion of this book and the second-most important thing a person should do, that is, get control of their weight by getting control of the numbers they're eating. Yes, that last meal you had was just a plate full of numbers. That, until now, you just looked at it as this or that, and so you are where you are because of it. The NCD will teach you to look at the meals and foods you are eating with greater insight and knowledge. When a nurse hangs an IV bag, she knows exactly what's in it and exactly what it will do when it goes into the body. So too do you need to think of eating in this same manner.

Up to this point, you have everything you need to determine if you are low on alkalinity, and if so, how to make the ABC Water as an alternative to increasing your alkalinity in lieu of eating more fruits and vegetables and less protein, i.e., in lieu of eating a vegetarian-style diet.

Should anyone tell you that maintaining your urine pH at exactly 7 is dangerous, ask them how it is that keeping the fluid exiting your kidneys at the same pH as plain water, a neutral pH, is dangerous. What is dangerous is walking around with excess acid in your system and depleted alkaline reserves and subjecting your kidney tissue to a pH near that of white vinegar.

Just as correcting the internal environment of your body can potentially have an effect of correcting a whole host of other health problems as a sort of byproduct of correcting the underlying condition, so it is with dropping fat. Excess body fat is implicated in many of today's health problems, and I don't need to list them all for you, you know, and you know if this is you. The Number Crunch Diet can help you take back the control you had as a small child, where the amount of calories that you consumed was in balance with the amount of calories that you used up.

I invented the NCD myself and have been using it and modifying it for over a decade. The features of the program you will not hear anywhere else as I made them up, I created them, they came to me in revelations as I dug deeper into the subject of fat loss, nutrition, meal making, and macronutrient percents.

Most diet plans differ in their macronutrient percents, or macros. We've touched on this already, Atkins being low carb high profat, and at the other end are the low-fat high-carb diets. The NCD is smack dab in the middle. You will be eating 500-calorie meals comprised of 40% carbohydrate, 30% fat, and 30% protein. The **Carbohydrate** provides you with energy required for the digestion of the meal, as well as energy to carry you to part of the way to your next meal. The **Fat** supplies your body with energy, cholesterol for steroid hormone synthesis, and lipid for the lipid membranes that encase the trillions of cells in your body. Unique to this diet plan is a never-before-seen way of regularly eating Omega-3 so that your cell membranes are flexible. Don't blame me if your skin becomes soft and youthful looking over time as you consume the NCD Flaxseed Shakes™ in this certain way that I explain in the recipe. Finally, the **Protein** component of the meals will break down into amino acids, becoming available for muscle tissue synthesis, for biochemical reactions related to all body functions, including metabolism, and to provide you with energy to sustain you to your next meal after your carbs have been used up.

This is why the other two extremes don't cut it for me. The high-carb 15%-protein diet doesn't contain sufficient protein to carry me to my next meal, hence I get moody. And the low-carb high-profat diet doesn't contain enough carbohydrate, hence I get moody. Both extremes are moody diets. They keep you from focusing on your life and instead have you focused on food. You eat to live, remember.

Already you should see how this makes perfect sense and is a healthy balanced approach to eating and weight control.

What makes this diet amazing is that ALL THE RECIPES HAVE BEEN DESIGNED TO CONTAIN 40% CARBS 30% FAT 30% PROTEIN AND 500 TOTAL CALORIES PER SERVING.

This is so effective in that it makes taking control of the numbers super easy. So if I have five meals a day, I've had 2500 calories. If I have four meals a day, I've had 2000 calories. Six meals a day, 3000 calories. A "Meal" is defined as 500 calories and a "Snack" is defined as 250 calories. If you have half a meal, 250 calories, that's a snack. So if one day I eat three meals and two snacks, I've had 2000 calories. Four meals and a snack, 2250 calories.

This makes tracking your calorie intake simple and easy, with the NCD Pre-Counted Meals™.

So I'm going to jump ahead a bit because I know you want to know, what you are going to be eating.

ANYTHING YOU WANT

With some exceptions, and that is, no empty calories, no chemicals, no poisons, no stimulants. How do you expect to maintain a healthy weight if your bloodstream and tissues are short on nutrition, if food additives and artificial sweeteners are toying with your bodily functions, and inflammation and hormonal upset is being brought on by trans, burnt, and omega-6 fats and high-fructose corn syrup, food dyes, and chemicals.

In the beginning you may find it difficult to break free from the hold that these foods have on you. You may find yourself with cravings that go on for days and perhaps weeks. My suggestion to you is this. Have it. However, sit in front of a mirror and have this book open at this page. Before each bite or drink of whatever it is that you are craving, read the above paragraph, take a bite if you must, and then look at yourself in the mirror as you chew.

Knowing the truth about what you are eating, you can't possibly eat it. Again, it comes back to that "truth setting you free" thing that Jesus talked about. This book will help you to look at food as an IV-infusion bag and how it affects your biology. Once you know the effects, the truth of it will set you free. Keep in mind you may have to read this material more than once to get it to sink in because your mind will want to skip over the parts you don't want to hear so you can continue on drinking badly and eating badly. Should you catch yourself tuning out, stop! That's your mind trying "not to hear it". Go back to the beginning and start over.

I believe there are valuable things written in many diet books but the reader didn't want to hear it, so their mind just tuned out as their eyes read over the words. I've done that.

This material has to sink in, in order for it to help you. So be aware of your mind playing that "tune out" game. Change is difficult for some people, it's as much a mental process of controlling the mind as it is an educational process of learning how to eat better.

I used to drink colas, with high-fructose corn syrup, the caramel color, sugar, phosphoric acid, caffeine, natural flavors, and zero nutrition. But, that was before I knew the truth about all of the damaging effects of those ingredients. Now that I know the truth, I'm free. I can sit across from someone who's drinking a glass of cola with crushed ice, or walk into a 7-Eleven and see the soft-drink fountain display, or walk down the soda-pop aisle at the grocery store, and have absolutely no desire for it. I'm free. But it was a process. Chemical addiction isn't just for street drugs, it's foods too. I gave-in a few times in the beginning, but as time passed it got easier and easier. It's a process, you have to wean yourself off if that food has a strong hold on you. I mean, you're literally dealing with chemicals.

The third main unique principle of the Number Crunch Diet is, you eat what you crave, and you don't eat what you don't crave.

The problem with so many diets is that they have you eating foods that you don't really want to eat. As time goes on, it gets worse and worse, until one day, you stop eating the foods on the diet meal plan and you go back to eating what you feel like eating.

The NCD says this. NEVER PUT A CALORIE IN YOUR MOUTH UNLESS IT'S REALLY WHAT YOU WANT. THINK ABOUT WHAT IT IS YOU WANT, AND THEN HAVE EXACTLY THAT.

What this does is shockingly amazing. It eliminates food cravings over time.

IT ELIMINATES FOOD CRAVINGS OVER TIME !!

You eat what you crave, and then you're good for a while. Then you eat what you crave again, a couple of weeks later, and you're good. Then you eat that same thing again, a few weeks or a month later. Then you eat it again a couple of months later. Then you eat it a half a year later. Then you eat it again a year later. Then you eat it again two years later. See, if you keep giving yourself what you crave, you no longer crave it after a while.

In fact, you can come to the point, where you don't crave any food at all. Which is what has occurred with me.

If carrot cake is your weakness, the NCD has a recipe meal that includes carrot cake. The recipe makes 10 servings, each with a $1/10^{th}$ portion of an entire carrot cake. If you have two servings a day of this meal, that's 500 calories x 2 = 1000 calories. You can still eat two more meals if your target is 2000 calories a day. At the end of 5 days, you've eaten an entire carrot cake. Your craving for carrot cake should be gone. If not, then make the recipe again, making 10 more meals. At the end of these 10 meals you will now have had two full carrot cakes. If your craving goes away but comes back next month, then make the recipe again, 10 meals and a full carrot cake. And if it comes back again the following month, make it again. That would be four full carrot cakes.

At a certain point, you are simply going to be bored with carrot cake and you're done with it. You might only make that recipe once every 1-2 years just to keep the craving at bay.

With the Number Crunch Diet, you eat what you crave, such that, over time, you no longer crave it.

You've had it so many times, you've gotten it out of your system.

You need to, GET IT OUT OF YOUR SYSTEM.

This doesn't happen by eating foods you don't particularly want.

EAT WHAT YOU CRAVE AND GET IT OUT OF YOUR SYSTEM.™

I've read almost 100 books in the past 13 years, and not one of them said this. This is completely new. And you heard it here first.

Eat What You Want and Get It Out Of Your System.™

This principle is the key to eliminating cravings.

I personally have eliminated my childhood desire for many baked goods this way. Cookies, cake, pudding, ice cream, I have no desire to eat any of these foods, and I merely have them once a year or once every two years just to keep any cravings from manifesting. But as a general rule, these childhood foods never enter my thoughts.

With the Number Crunch Diet plan, you eat the foods you crave, incorporated into a meal, so that you don't gain weight. As in the carrot cake example, I ate an entire carrot cake in 5 days, eating $1/10^{th}$ of the cake with my breakfast meal, and $1/10^{th}$ of the cake with my lunch meal, and I did that for 5 days. There was no weight gain because the carrot cake was the fat and carb portion of my meal. I added a side of chicken breast for protein, cooked in a skillet with a flour salt and pepper coating, and Mmm. Party time!

I typically eat 2500 calories a day, so if I had wanted to, I could have eaten the carrot-cake skillet-chicken meal at 07:00, 11:00, 14:00, 17:00, 20:00, and not gained weight. But that would have been way too much carrot cake, even for me.

Now you do have to pay attention to sugar, and the carrot-cake skillet-chicken is a treat meal, but the purpose is to eat it and get it out of your system. If there are treats that you like to eat, incorporate them into meals, eat them, and get them out of your system.

INCORPORATE TREATS INTO MEALS, THEN EAT THEM AND GET THEM OUT OF YOUR SYSTEM.

This is the #1 foundational principle of the NCD.
You eat what you crave and get it out of your system.

EAT IT, AND GET IT OUT OF YOUR SYSTEM™

Gradually, over time, you will choose nutritious foods over treat foods and treat foods will only be a small part of your diet.

There is more to come in the following chapters, but this introduces you to a few of the key aspects of the NCD, and how it differs from all the other plans. I used this plan to lower my weight from 172 lbs to 145 lbs and add about 15 lbs of muscle in the process, which bodybuilders claim you can't build muscle and lose fat at the same time. Well, I did. At the end of about five months, I had visible veins and very thin skin on my lower abs, essentially no love handles, and the veins in my forearms and upper arms were so close to the surface it was scary-freaky. At that point, muscle gains had plateaued and that's when I decided to try that "Bulking" thing bodybuilders talk about. I tell you this only to let you know that I do the program myself, and the calorie-counting principle that I've come up with, whereby you count calories by counting Pre-Counted Meals™, is a unique feature to the NCD. With complete control of the numbers, you can work the NCD in any direction you want to go, weight loss, weight gain, or weight maintenance.

CHAPTER 38

FOOD CRAVINGS

I'm going to start with a discussion of food cravings because I've made some interesting discoveries about how to eliminate them. Discoveries that, if you should hear them anywhere else, they took them from this publication. This chapter is unique, new, never-heard-before information for dealing with food cravings. How do I know? The insights came to me as Divine understanding as I searched for the answers. Just like how one would write an original song, I created these original methods of overcoming food cravings. I emphasize this because so much of what's out there is rehashed repackaged material with a slight variation. New, unique, original material is hard to come by and worth its weight in 'gold'.

Top-of-the-list, cravings for Ice Cream. If this is you, I can relate. At one time in my life I stocked four different flavors of ice cream in my freezer, French Vanilla, Chocolate, Vanilla Fudge Swirl, and Mint Chocolate Chip. Is your mouth watering? Mine's not. I have not purchased a container of ice cream in more than ten years. I can walk down the freezer aisle and look at all those flavors and feel nothing. This can be you too.

How did I come to get off of my addiction to ice cream, yes, addiction. I had a bowl every day, and I never had less-than two flavors in stock. AND, I knew I was addicted but I just couldn't see a way out. Ice cream was part of my childhood upbringing, and, as a young adult, I just continued eating it on a regular basis.

At 35 years of age, I couldn't remember a time when I didn't eat ice cream. Ice cream was as much a part of me as my arms, legs, head, and soul.

So here's what I discovered. My body really wanted milk.

If you crave ice cream, your body is asking for milk.™

The same is true for ketchup.

If you crave french fries with ketchup, your body wants tomatoes.™

French fries your weakness?

If you crave french fries, your body wants potatoes.™

Do you know what pica is? Pica is a condition where a young developing child eats dirt. Do you think the child likes the taste of dirt so he or she just decides to eat dirt? Of course not. The body's intelligence is searching for nutrients, in this case, minerals.

My sister adopted a child from an orphanage overseas and he ate dirt.

Cribbing has alternate definitions, but it is used to describe a horse chewing and eating wood, or a baby chewing on the wooden poles of its crib.

What is going on in these cases? Do these children have a dirt or wood deficient diet? Of course not.

They are eating something in order to get something they're missing.

Ketchup – you're missing tomatoes.
French Fries – you're missing potatoes.
Ice Cream – you're missing milk.

What if much of the food you eat over and over again, and overeat, what if, your body's searching for something it needs?

Well, not "what if", THAT'S EXACTLY WHAT'S HAPPENING.

Your body's not stupid.   We just don't pay attention to its communication. Or we don't understand its communication.

So, when I started drinking more milk, specifically, one quart of milk a day, I noticed I didn't have a desire for ice cream.

THERE'S YOUR ANSWER RIGHT THERE.

You heard it here first.   YOUR CRAVING FOR ICE CREAM CAN BE ELIMINATED BY DRINKING MILK.™

Now, one or two 8oz glasses here-and-there isn't going to cut it. You're deficient. You need milk therapy! I went from one quart a day to two gallons a week, and often, two gallons from Monday to Friday. My aggressive milk treatment curbed my craving for ice cream almost overnight. I quickly saw the connection.

By drinking two gallons of milk a week, I stopped buying ice cream completely. I would walk down the ice-cream aisle and my autopilot program would say "oh, I should buy ice cream" and I would stop, snap myself out of autopilot, and then my next thought would be, "I don't really want ice cream."

I was beginning to override my autopilot and listen to my Divine Intelligence. Before you eat something, you have to check with your Divine Intelligence. Ask it what it wants. By Divine Intelligence, I am referring to the internal Divine Intelligence that runs your body. You don't have to tell your heart to beat at a perfect rhythm 60 times a minute. You don't have to tell your finger to heal from a paper cut. You don't have to tell your Divine Intelligence anything. IT'S THE BOSS. Your Divine Intelligence operating your interior is the boss. It's in charge. It knows exactly what to do on the inside of you.

If you want to drive your car across town, you are in charge. That's exterior. That's the outer you. For most of us, this is the only you you know. Today, let me introduce you to the other you. The inner you. The guy running the inside. Your Divine Intelligence.

You, the outer you, is not the boss of your interior functions.

It's a bit hard at first for the ego to admit that it's not the boss of everything about you. But it's not. You have an inner Boss.

So, applying this to eating. YOU NEED TO CHECK WITH YOUR DIVINE INTELLIGENCE AND SEE WHAT IT WANTS.™

Instead, we let our exterior make the choices and we give our body whatever our exterior body sees, craves, looks at, or wants.

FROM THIS DAY FORWARD, YOU NEED TO MAKE ALL OF YOUR FOOD CHOICES FROM THE INSIDE.

Not from the outside. I want I want I want. Because it's going to make me feel good.

Eating is about supplying your body with nutrition. It's not about feeling good.

If you need to eat something, or smoke something, or drink something, to make you feel happy, then you are compensating.

Compensating. Compensating. Compensating for what?

Only you can discover that.

Were you neglected as a child? Do you, as an adult, look for other people to love you? Your spouse, your children, your friends. Have people or someone been cruel to you in the past, or currently? Cruelty happens everywhere, especially if you are gentle and nice. The world hates gentle and nice. It's weak, they say. This is why they murdered Jesus Christ, he was a nice guy. What did he do that the people of his day wanted to kill him so badly? In the New Testament it describes Jesus going here and there and then it finishes with "and he healed them".   The guy healed people everywhere he went. And yet, the "world" hated him.

So buck up my friend. It is possible to be gentle and nice, and not let people, sadists, walk all over you. If they crucify you in the end, so be it. At least you were your own person.

Whatever feeling you have that is controlling your eating, you need to identify it, see it, look at it, and say to it, "Game's over, I know what you've been doing to me."

This is not a psychology book, but food addiction is the topic, and food addiction, like any other addiction, plays out in your body, through your mind, from prior trauma.   There's a Pavlovian Conditioned Response going on if you "have to" have chocolate, or you "have to" have wine, or you "have to" have french fries. And there's a chemical component too. It's been said, that the mental component, a fear of hurt, that overweight people tend to have, is why they build a wall of protection around themselves, through food. If this is you, don't feel bad, the lean person is doing the same thing, but just using a pill, or a bottle, or a credit card, or any of the dozens of other ways people compensate.

The solution for all addictions, including food addiction, is, to stop allowing yourself to decide your choices and let your internal Divine Intelligence make your choices.

You are in the driver's seat if you need to drive across town. That's external. But when it comes to your internals, i.e., eating and nutrition, get out of the driver's seat and hand the steering wheel over to your Divine Intelligence.

CHAPTER 39

Food Cravings Part 2

The fourth method for eliminating food cravings is…

Fourth? What were one, two and three? You tell me. I didn't number them on purpose because I want to see if you are paying attention, perhaps even taking some notes, or are you just skimming on through. If you skim through this book, you will get to the end and be the exact same person as you were when you started.

For those of you who are making notes in the margin, have a highlighter in your hand, and are reading only one of these chapters at a time, so that the material sinks in, I applaud you.

For the skimmers, you might as well just close this book now. You are not going to make any changes in your lifestyle or eating behavior.

Someone I once worked with gave me the diet book, *The Whole Truth*. She said she was finished reading it and that I could have it. I read it, my usual way. I underlined and highlighted important points, I made notes in the margin, and I tabbed the chapters so that it would be easy to find information later on if I needed to reread something. But there's more. I take cardstock, cut it to the size of the book, and I tape extra pages into the back of the book. This is key, so listen closely.

Now, as I read the information in the book, I come across new information.   That new information combines with the stored information on the hard disk of my brain, and bingo! Revelation. The light comes on. NEW UNDERSTANDING comes to me. New Knowledge. So it is, on these extra blank pages, is where I write my revelations. Hence, the material in this book is NEW material. Information that I read, combines with information that I know, to create completely new insights and information.

If you have kids, teach them to read books this way.

So, back to work and I tell my coworker thanks for the book, Andrea Beaman has an interesting personal testimony and I started to talk about the book. My coworker had a blank look on her face. So I then said, "I thought you read the book." She said, "I did." I thought to myself, you did but you don't remember any of it. The point is, skimming through the chapters is not reading. You will be the same person doing the same things you were doing ten years ago. It's like the high-school reunion and almost everybody's the same, just older. You should be learning as you journey through your life. Changing. Growing. Evolving.

My goal is to help you and that means, that yes, I have to tell you how to read a book. So go tape some pages to the back of this book. Use this book, in conjunction with what you already know, to write down revelations that come to you. These revelations are your answers to becoming a better you.

#1 Eat the food you crave and get it out of your system.
I used the example of the carrot cake. If you want carrot cake eat carrot cake, but incorporate it into a meal. If you want carrot cake, then DO NOT eat rice cakes. You don't want rice cakes. You don't eat foods you don't want, just because you think they are going to help you lose weight. You are going to lose weight by getting control of the numbers you're eating, and by getting rid of food cravings. You do this by eating them, incorporated into a meal, and repeating the recipe again and again, until one day, you are bored with carrot cake. You can look at pizza and say, I'm

done with pizza. You can look at potato chips and say, no thanks.
You can look at macaroni salad and say, nah been there done that. I
can honestly tell you that I have eliminated all of my food cravings,
and eat a very clean nutritious diet. If I see something that gets my
attention, I come up with a meal recipe, incorporate that food into
the meal, make eight or however many servings, eat them and get it
out of my system. If I want to do it again next week, fine, I do it
again. The key is. You incorporate it into a meal. You don't eat
the meal and then have the cheesecake. That's not how it works.
That's what put the extra weight on in the first place.

#2 You don't eat chemicals or poisons. Well you said you had
carrot cake. The Trader Joe's carrot cake is almost exactly like my
mother's homemade carrot cake recipe; sugar, not HFCS, carrots,
the second ingredient is carrots!, amazing, soybean oil, okay, flour,
eggs, walnuts, cream cheese, butter, baking soda, bicarbonate!, salt,
cinnamon, pure vanilla, not the fake vanilla flavoring, and
modified corn starch, okay. Carrots are the second most abundant
ingredient, plus real cream cheese, real walnuts, real vanilla, real
butter, not margarine or hydrogenated fat.   Soybean oil
occasionally is not going to kill me. Soybean oil regularly,
absolutely not. This recipe and the NCD Coleslaw™ dressing are
the only two times I eat soybean oil. It would be better if it read
organic soybean oil, but 90% of the soybeans grown are GMO,
genetically modified, so they don't qualify for being organic.

So, the NCD says you can use packaged food if it's a good product.
And there are good products out there, especially at the healthfood
store, you just have to read the label. Everything on the label
should be a food. The TJs carrot cake is made from other foods.

A chemical or poison are things like, HFCS high-fructose corn
syrup, margarine, hydrogenated oil, or worse, partially-
hydrogenated oil, or still worse, burnt deep-fried oil, caramel color,
sodium benzoate preservative, dyes, yellow #5, red #40, blue #1,
all dyes are out, no dyes period, MSG, glycols, polysorbates,
basically anything that you don't recognize as a food. The major
ones are HFCS, hydrogenated oil, dyes, and chemical additives.

Nitrites should be avoided, but the NCD Ham & Pea Soup™ does use ham with nitrites on the label, but again, occasionally or rarely is acceptable. Nitrites in Moderation, absolutely not.

So if you are hooked on a particular food, say, powdered mini donuts, sit facing a mirror with this book and the ingredients label in front of you and read the ingredients, look at this book, and take a bite of the donut, if you must.

The theory behind this technique is, that a normal mentally-healthy adult cannot intentionally and knowingly do harm to themselves. The book is the truth that you know, the label shows the ingredients, and the mirror is you seeing you harm yourself. You can't do it. I wouldn't be surprised if you spit the donut out and throw the whole thing in the trash and then take it outside to the trash bin and discard it away from you and away from your house.

Now if you eat the whole donut and think "I don't care", and there are many self-destructive people like this in society, well, I think psychiatrists have a name for people who knowingly do harm to themselves with a complete disregard for the consequences.

A normal healthy adult will see the truth, and look at themselves, be disgusted, and turn over a new leaf. You're free.

Don't feel bad. We've all done it and many many people continue to poison themselves daily, one bite at a time. I already told you the ingredients in pepsi, and I drank gallons of that stuff every month for a number of years.

Kevin Trudeau in his book, *Natural Cures They Don't Want You To Know About*, exposed the dirty little secret about the food industry. "They put chemicals in the food to make you addicted to the product."

I have in front of me a Wendy's Nutrition Ingredients Guide, and I'm not singling out Wendy's, I used to eat there once if not twice a week. I also have Nutrition Ingredients Guides from McDonald's and Jack-In-The-Box, they're all basically the same. Here are some ingredients that are jumping out at me off the page, Autolyzed Yeast Extract, Spices, Artificial Color, Natural Flavor, Disodium Inosinate (flavor enhancer), EDTA (flavor protector), Sodium Benzoate, Yellow 5 and 6, Azodicarbonamide (dough conditioner), Caramel Color, BHT, Artificial Flavor, Guanylate (flavor enhancer), Corn Syrup, Sodium Erythorbate (buffering agent), Cottonseed Oil, Calcium Propionate (preservative), and on and on. The list of chemicals, dyes, colors, flavorings, stabilizers, conditioners, etc., is endless. I encourage you to explore this on your own. If it's not a food, it's a chemical. A chemical addiction.

The Number Crunch Diet says that you have to make your own meals if you want to be successful at taking control of your weight by taking control of the numbers.

It is possible to find good-quality restaurant food, but you have to look for it and you will likely be paying $15-20 for one meal. If you took $20 a day times 30 days, that's $600. You could purchase nearly all organic food from a healthfood store with $600 a month. Plus restaurants overcook the proteins and then the protein portion of the meal is semi-worthless.

Start by making one NCD recipe per month. It may divide into 8 or 12 or 16 meals, depending on the recipe. So if you eat two of the recipe meals per day, that would be 6 days, if you made 12 meals. Then, make the recipe again the next week to master the procedure and speed up your time in the kitchen. Next month try a new recipe and repeat the process. At the end of 12 months you will have added 12 NCD meal recipes to your meal-making repertoire. At this point you could be eating 75% homemade meals and 25% packaged, processed, fastfood, and restaurant meals. Add another 12 recipes during the second year, and before long, 100% of your diet will be from homemade meals you prepare yourself.

#3   #3   #3   Come on, what's number three? This is the most important one. Go back to the previous chapter and read it again if you don't remember.

DIVINE INTELLIGENCE

You, the you on the outside, no longer decides what you are going to eat. Before each meal, and as you plan to make meals for the upcoming days, you pause and ask yourself, "What do I want?" You ask your Divine Intelligence, your internal you, what it wants based on what it needs. You have no idea if you are low on zinc or copper. You have no idea if you need lycopene or zeaxanthin, plant color nutrients. You have no idea if you need lysine, or carnitine, or alpha-lipoic acid, or any of the hundreds, if not thousands of tiny nutrient molecules that scientists haven't even discovered yet. But your Divine Intelligence knows. So #3 is, let your Divine Intelligence guide your eating. If you do this, one day you will be so well nourished that when you go to ask yourself what you want, the answer comes back, "Nothing Really". Imagine your body being so stocked up with nutrition that you don't really feel like eating anymore. You just do it because you know you need to provide your body with a steady supply of proteins fats carbohydrates and nutrients to keep it running and in tiptop condition. This should be your long-term goal.

So if you didn't already do so in the previous chapter, then do it now. From this moment forward, my Divine Intelligence makes all of my food choices. Ask it, and pause, the answer will come to you. The other way that it can happen is by interruption. You are going through your day and your DI grabs your attention and says, "Hey, how about some Brazil nuts, they're lookin' real good right now." Or you might hear, "I need milk again, we're out in here." Or you just get a strong urge to eat cooked carrots, or green beans, or chicken. Listen and comply. If you want your body to work for you, you had better work for your body. So if you catch yourself buying food that YOU want, the external you, that's a NCD rule breaker. From this moment forward the internal you is the boss of what you eat. Emotional eating, eating to get a FEELING or to suppress a bad feeling, or to lift your mood, or to help you cope with life, this is where you went wrong to begin with. Look for better ways to cope with life and separate your feelings from your eating, and leave the food choices up to your Divine Intelligence.

CHAPTER 40

Food Cravings Part 3

Okay, we didn't get to #4 in that last chapter, but I think it helped to solidify the one, two and three.

The fourth method…

By the way, if anyone reading this knows someone who knows someone that's got a television show, ask them to have me on as a guest. I could talk for two hours on this subject and alkalinity and just be getting warmed up.

#4   Stay Full. Now that doesn't mean stuffed full all the time, it means, DON'T GO MORE THAN FOUR HOURS WITHOUT EATING! You see, if you are not hungry, you don't have food cravings. However, if you haven't eaten in 4.5 to 5 or 5.5 hours, you are going to be wanting to eat anything and everything you see. The NCD rule for meal frequency is, every 2-4 hours, being very careful not to go beyond 4.

Women who postpone eating just put the people around them walking on thin ice. You women out there that take your lunch break at your 6th hour of work, practically at the end of your shift, do the rest of us a favor and go eat. If this is you, you have no idea how grumpy and miserable you are because you've been doing this to yourself for so long. Four Hours. No longer than four hours without eating. Even if it's half a meal, 250 calories. You need food to function, so stop putting off eating and depriving yourself, you're never going to lose fat that way anyway, and it's been proven over and over.

For example, if you are a 5 foot 6 inch 165 lb woman and you need to drop some weight, your day might look like this.
06:00 Up
07:00 500 calories
3 hrs
10:00 250 calories
2 hrs
12:00 500 calories
3 hrs
15:00 250 calories
2 hrs
17:00 500 calories
3 hrs
20:00 250 calories
2 hrs
22:00 Bed

This is fantastic. You are eating six times a day, every day. Your total calories are 2250 per day, which is likely the number of calories you need to maintain your weight. This person is eating all day. Good. She's maintaining a steady supply of energy, glucose, protein, fats, and nutrients, and should not be hungry. This person should be going through her day feeling focused, emotionally stable, and productive. She is eating at regular intervals, spaced apart, and calorie balanced. Nothing two hours before bed, should ensure that she doesn't gain weight.

If this person wants to lose fat, then reduce your daily calories by 250 or 500. Never reduce your calories by more than 20%. In other words, always eat calories equal to at least 80% of your daily maintenance calorie requirement.

In this example, 2250 x 0.80 is 1800 calories. It's okay to round this to 1750 to make the numbers easier. The 80% rule is a guide, and 50 calories is not all that significant. The point is, you don't cut your calorie intake in half or by 60 or 70%. Your body just goes into starvation mode, and you can't lose fat in starvation mode. Recall how we looked at the concept of Homeostasis, and how your body doesn't want to shift from where it is currently, and so you have to trick your body's homeostatic mechanism by implementing changes mildly, "smoothly". Cutting calories by more than 20% is not going to fool your homeostatic mechanism and three-months later you'll be right back where you started.

So this person could cut 250 calories from her daily diet or at the most, cut 500 calories from her daily diet. Or she could do a mixed version, MWF cut 500, TRSaSu cut 250, where R=Thurrrrsday. Cutting 500 calories per day will result in a loss of 1 lb of pure fat from her body each week. She could also alternate, week one cut 500 per day seven-days-a-week, week two cut 250 per day seven-days-a-week. This approach is safe and gradual. Slow and steady wins the race (it's trite, but it's true).

So where is she going to cut? Well, her 17:00 500-calorie dinner could be cut to 250. That's not hard. If she wanted to lose fat a little faster, omit the 20:00 250-calorie snack, and make your 17:00 500-calorie meal the last meal of your day. This would result in no eating five hours before bed. Believe me, if she sticks to this, she will be waking up every single morning thinner and thinner. All she has to do is cut out that one 20:00 evening snack and she will be losing fat daily. KITCHEN CLOSED AT FIVE. If you can close that kitchen at 5pm, five hours before bed, you will easily lose and maintain your weight. The question becomes, can you go five hours in the evening without eating? That's the tricky part.

Now, there are times when you can break the NCD Four-Hour Rule™ for meal frequency, and that is when it occurs at the end of your day. If your last meal of 500cal is at 17:00, then four hours later is 21:00, and you are going to be winding it down to be in bed by 22:00. The Four-Hour Rule applies to the busy productive part of your day. Closing the kitchen three, four, and even five hours before bed is an excellent way to lose fat and maintain your weight.

In our example, if she makes her last meal at 17:00 and has to go five hours without food, this may not be a problem because she's eaten five times that day already, and her 17:00 meal is 500 calories. Suppose this meal is the NCD Chicken Caesar Salad™ which includes an english muffin with strawberry jam, she may be completely satisfied until bedtime. Meals that are 40% carbs 30% fat 30% protein and 500 calories can last me 5 to 5.5 and even 6 hours. They are very satisfying. Now I don't go 5, 5.5, or 6 hours without eating, but the point is, no other combination of numbers will provide such a sustaining effect. This is why the Number Crunch Diet is called the Number Crunch Diet. All the meals are number crunched to 40 30 30 and 500 calories.

If she eats this type of meal at 17:00 she will have no problem making it to her 22:00 bedtime. So all she has to do is omit the 250 calories at 20:00 and have nothing five hours before bed. As the fat comes off and she starts to feel hungry in the evening, there are NCD Calorie-Free Vegetables™ that a person can have to carry them to their next meal or to bedtime, and these will be addressed later.

After a couple of months, she can mix it up a bit. Have the 20:00 snack of 250 calories, but cut 250 calories from breakfast and 250 calories from lunch. So 250 250 250 250 500 250 = 1750 calories. She still gets to eat six times a day every two to three hours, plus she gets to eat in the evening 250 calories two hours before bed, but she's cutting back her breakfast and lunch meals from 500 to 250. As long as she stays calm, this will work for her. It's a 500 calorie a day cut, but she gets to eat six times a day all day, right up until two hours before bed.

She could do that for a few weeks to speed up some fat loss, and then switch to a milder approach by adding back 250 calories to either the breakfast or the lunch, and she will still come in at 250 calories less per day and feeling like she's always eating and never hungry.

You can play with the numbers any way you want. Just don't go more than four hours without eating or you risk becoming hungry, and hunger spells disaster.

Also, if you are going to cut calories, stick to cutting in increments of 250 and 500. It makes it easier to keep track of. If you want to cut your calories by 350 per day, then use the mixed method, MWF cut 500, TRSaSu cut 250. This averages to a cut of 357 calories per day, or about 350, and three-quarters of a pound of body fat per week.

One pound of body fat is equal to 3500 calories. Therefore, cutting 250 calories a day will have you losing half-a-pound per week. Cutting 350 per day, three-quarters of a pound of fat per week. And a 500 per day cut will result in one whole pound of fat off your body each week. It only takes 2-3-4 pounds of fat loss to start feeling thinner. Then once you've got the ball rolling, just stick with it until you reach your goal weight.

Follow the NCD 80/20 Rule™ when cutting calories, that is, don't cut your calories by more than 20% of your maintenance requirement, or said the other way, always eat at least 80% of your maintenance calorie requirement.

For me personally, I eat 2500 calories a day for maintenance, five meals a day, 500x5=2500. If I want to cut fat, I have many choices. I can eat 500x3 plus 250x2 = 2000 calories per day. Or I can eat four meals of 500 calories each spaced four-hours apart. Or I can throw in a workout 30-45 minutes a day, raising my calorie requirement to 3000 per day while continuing to eat 2500 per day. If I want to add size, I can work out 30-45 minutes a day, eat 3000 calories M-Sa, and do a carb-load on Sunday, FFS Fat Free Sunday. I could also eat half a meal, 250 calories, before bed, so that I wake up with bigger fuller muscles. It's all numbers. Weight Loss or Weight Gain, when you control the numbers, you control the desired result.

CHAPTER 41

Food Cravings Part 4

Now, before we move to the fifth and final technique for eliminating food cravings, let me ask that you not take anything that I have written or expressed and twist it. When I say, Fat Loss Is A Numbers Game, and that, It's All About The Numbers, of course I am fully informed of the many other conditions that affect fat loss or muscle gain.

If you have yeast, you'll need to get free of your yeast or you will have a hard time eliminating sugar and carb cravings from your diet and hence the numbers game isn't going to work well for you. If you have parasites/worms, and this is not just an underdeveloped country problem, pet owners are often infected with parasites, and those with unclean lifestyles or habits, these people will have a difficult time losing weight. People with a sluggish thyroid will have difficulty losing weight. If you're lacking in normal healthy gut flora you are going to have a harder time losing weight.

People who simply don't chew their food will find themselves eating more because they can't remember eating their last meal that was only 30 minutes prior but they failed to chew it and enjoy it and now they are looking to eat again, these people will have a hard time losing weight. If I am speaking to you, you need to slow down and chew every mouthful of food before swallowing, in fact, if this is you, I want you to DOUBLE CHEW everything you eat. This means, you chew your mouthful of food, but before you swallow it, you bring it to the front of your mouth again and chew it all a second time. This NCD Double Chew™ technique will have you eating slower, and quite possibly, half as much food. Your stomach will signal that it's full and you will put the remainder of your meal back in the refrigerator, finishing it as a snack 2-3 hours later. For some of you, this may be all you need to do to lose weight. But this applies to everyone. We all eat too fast. You know, other cultures around the world take an hour or more to eat dinner. After a bite of food, they put their fork down, chew, pause, and then pick their fork up again for the next bite. If we aren't finished a meal in ten minutes, we feel like we are going too slow, stopping and dying, when the truth is, those fast meals are killing you. Slow down. Double Chew and Put The Fork Down.

A good habit to get into doing is to Pray before each meal. It can just be a simple few words of thanksgiving for the fact that you have food to eat. What it does is, it places a line between what you were just doing, say working, and what you are now about to do, eating. The NCD Pray Before Meals™ changes the physiology of your body from external, (work and do activities), to internal, (digestive activities). Many times I have eaten in a rushed setting and the food just sat there. Then I would eat more food to get the meal I just ate to move, when all I need to do was to stop, pray, allow my physiology to change gears, and then eat.

For the slow thyroid person, if your TSH, thyroid stimulating hormone test, is greater-than or equal to 3, 3 being the middle of the normal range, your thyroid is already getting sluggish. The TSH normal range goes up to about 6, so 6.1 would flag high, but at that point you are already stage-two sluggish. You want your TSH to be 2, 2.5, 3 at the most. To fix this, do Sweat Cardio. Wake that thyroid up and get that whole hormonal loop moving with movement. Your thyroid's become sluggish, because your lifestyle's become sluggish. Hypo means too little, too low, too slow. Pick up the pace of your lifestyle and your thyroid will follow. It won't hurt to supplement with iodine, 150ug a day is the minimum, and check your body temperature. I have selfcare protocols for both of these so stay tuned!

For the yeast person, cut your carbs and sugars to zip, to as low as you can. This is where you need radical. Do the Atkins diet for a month or more to deplete your sugar stores and starve that yeast out of your body. A person with yeast is more than likely carrying around extra fat. In fact, I will go as far as to say that if you are obese, you most likely have yeast in your intestinal tract, and possibly elsewhere. Your Internal Environment plays a key role here. The yeast person needs to get that urine pH up from 5 to 6 to 7. Fermented acidic foods are where yeast love to thrive. Is your body's internal environment mimicking that of fermented foods? I hope not. Raising your urine pH out of that vinegar range may be all you need. If you have yeast and can't seem to get rid of it, check your urine pH.

In addition to maintaining my urine pH at 7, for additional yeast prevention I take Oil of Oregano, Wild Mediterranean Oregano Leaf with 70% carvacrol, the active ingredient. I take one gel cap once or twice a week as my anti-yeast, anti-fungus, anti-mycoplasma insurance plan.

For the parasite and worm person, you need to first identify the source and get rid of it. If it's dirty living, clean and sanitize, if you garden, bleach your fingernails, if you are around pets or animals you are constantly exposing yourself to the "things" they have. Deworming might work, but it might not. Once you've cleaned up or removed the source, then it's time to remove them from your body. Back to www.drclarkstore.com for the Green Black Walnut Hull tincture, or better yet, do the full 17-day parasite cleanse with the Cloves and the Wormwood.

The vitamin- and mineral-deficient person needs to supplement. If you've ever been told that you have a magnesium deficiency or an iron deficiency, or any mineral deficiency, then you can assume you are deficient in ALL minerals, and likely vitamins as well. A nutrient-depleted diet means you've not been getting enough of ALL nutrients. Supplement to get your levels back into the normal range and get your body working optimally again. So, yes, fat loss is more than a numbers game.

#5   The last method for eliminating food cravings is, to eat something similar instead.   For example, if you are hooked on Kentucky Fried Chicken, you will never unhook yourself as long as you keep going back there to eat it.   So, to unhook yourself, you are going to make a similar version, but you control the ingredients and the portion size and calories.   There was a time when I could eat KFC several times a month.   A whole bucket of chicken, or a 9-piece box, not a problem.   I could eat 4-5-6 pieces and still be wanting more a couple of hours later.   This was not normal.

So when I read Kevin Trudeau's book and how he harped on the fact that food companies, manufacturers, and restaurants, put chemicals in their food to make you addicted to their product, I knew this was happening to me.   You will never get free if you keep going back to the pusher for your fix.   You've got to have a quitting plan, the NCD Quitting Plan™.

You will need to find a similar meal that you can have that is healthy and free of chemicals, so that you can enjoy eating the food you want without deprivation.   Just cutting out KFC chicken didn't work for me.   I had to find a substitute.   And I did.

The NCD Skillet Chicken™ recipe is a formulation that I can eat over and over again and never get bored, but I don't overeat it.   And it's just as good as the one I was addicted to.   Better actually.   Less stimulating.   And less fattening.

To a 16oz glass jar, like the kind you bought at sks-bottle.com, add 180g of flour.   Now right there you say, "What measuring cup do I use?"   Just get used to measuring your ingredients by weight, using a scale, instead of by volume, using measuring cups.   Weight is more accurate and creates fewer dishes to wash.   You place the 16oz jar on the scale and press "tare" to zero it.   Now, scoop in flour until it says 180 grams.   If you bought the S&F scale you can toggle back-and-forth from ounces to grams with the touch of a button.   Next, add 17g of finely ground black pepper, and then 32g of Lawry's Seasoned Salt No MSG.   Be sure to buy the seasoned salt that says "No MSG" on the front.   Although it does contain

"Natural Flavors" which is basically a code word for addictive chemicals.

Do you remember the ingredients from the Wendy's Nutrition Guide?   Do you recall reading Disodium Inosinate (flavor enhancer)? Remember Accent, the "spice", in the white container with the red trim, the cylinder-shaped container, Accent, the flavor enhancer, Accent, that has one ingredient on the label, monosodium glutamate, MSG. Disodium Inosinate is doing the same thing to your physiology, it's just a different chemical name.

So the healthier, less chemically-risky version of the NCD Skillet Chicken™ is to substitute seasalt for the Lawry's Seasoned Salt. I have switched to the seasalt version and it tastes almost the same. However the seasoned salt does make the chicken taste more like KFC. So, in the beginning, to get off the KFC chicken, use the NCD Skillet Chicken™ with the Lawry's Seasoned Salt, and then get off the Lawry's Seasoned Salt by switching to seasalt. So it's like a Two Step Chemical Addiction Program.

Look, food cravings are no different than cigarette cravings or alcohol cravings or drug cravings. Chemicals work the same way regardless of where you put them. And Kevin Trudeau already exposed the fact that it's in the foods we eat, hidden under "Natural Flavorings" and "Spices".

Whenever I see either of these two words on a label, I insert the phrase, "Chemicals That Make Me Addicted To Their Product".

This is why the NCD #2 Craving Eliminator™, no chemicals or poisons, is so critically important. They have you hooked.

If you can, shop at the healthfood store, these companies disclose everything. Some food companies include so much writing and information on their product that they barely have room on the label for the product name. This is excellent. Contrast this with breakfast cereals. What do you see? All name, cartoon pictures, decals, and very little about what you are actually eating and nothing about how it will assist your Divine Intelligence to do its job.

One way to quickly get healthy is to start today by eating all of your food from a healthfood store. My local healthfood store, Lassen's Health Foods, is excellent. I very rarely see a food label with the words "Natural Flavoring" "high-fructose corn syrup" or "monosodium glutamate" on a product in their store. In fact, many companies refuse to use general words like "Spices" but rather they will list every individual spice they use.

Why is it that your average everyday supermarket has so many ingredients on their shelves that the consumer has no idea what they mean?

Why is it that the healthfood store has almost none of these same chemical ingredients?

Every time you spend a dollar you vote. I encourage you to begin today to vote with your dollars. Support Heinz mustard for removing "Natural Flavoring" from its label, and replacing it with the words, "salt, turmeric, and paprika", words that are foods, that people can understand. Boycott French's, who, at the time of this writing, is still hiding behind "Natural Flavoring" on their mustard label. Buy as many of your groceries from your healthfood store as you can. The food manufacturers that supply Lassen's Health Foods are some of the brightest, honest, most noble companies on the planet. Support them with as much of your dollars as you can and vote out the food companies that are putting chemicals in the food they make. Flavor enhancers are addictive chemicals, having the same effect as any other addictive chemical. Just say "No!" to Natural Flavoring Enhancing Drugs.

So whatever foods you find yourself addicted to, maybe it's buffalo wings, well, buy some chicken and marinate it in tabasco with some butter, then bake them. Whatever it is, find a substitute that you can make yourself from real foods, and switch to eating that.

CHAPTER 42

RECAP

So let's review our NCD Food Craving Rules™.

1. Eat the foods you crave and get them out of your system.
2. Don't eat chemicals or poisons, any word that is not a food.
3. Check with your Divine Intelligence when deciding what to eat.
4. Stay "full", never going more than four hours without eating.
5. To break addiction to a food, make something similar yourself.

You know, I've read dozens of books on diet and can't think of one of them that ever mentioned food addictions, outside of *Natural Cures They Don't Want You To Know About*. Well, Dr. Mercola's *No Grain Diet* has a tapping method, the Emotional Freedom Technique, but it's going to take more than tapping to break you free from food chemicals.

What I've given you in these first five chapters of the Number Crunch Diet should have your head spinning. This information should be shattering your world. If you read this, and read it thoroughly, you should be a changed person. You are halfway free already just by seeing the truth. Now, the rest is up to you.

What are you going to do differently? Perhaps, if you've never shopped at your local healthfood store, maybe you will drive over there and walk up-and-down the aisles and look at all the amazing products. Pick them up and read the labels. The first thing you will see when you walk into Lassen's is a wall full of books. Books. Information. Education. Insider Information. There was a time when the first thing you saw when you walked into Safeway were baked goods; pastries, cakes, pies, all fattening chemical-laden junk. Now they have fresh fruit and vegetable displays in the front, much better.

Maybe you will turn the product around and read the back, read everything on the label, read every word on every label of every product that you buy. In the 1990s, I was the only person who stood in an aisle reading the back of the label. Not one person was doing this back then. I stood out. Now, I often see people doing what I do, and that is, I reach for the product on the shelf, and as I bring it towards me, I rotate my hand 180 degrees. Try it right where you are right now. Imagine a shelf in front of you, reach forward with your arm, take the item, and as you bring it towards you, rotate your hand 180 degrees. Never mind the front. Read the back.

After all, I'm not there to buy cartoon characters, logos, decals, and pictures, I'm there to find nutrients that my Divine Intelligence needs to run my body. It tells me what to eat, and I listen to its subtle communications. But I already know a lot of what it needs already. It wants milk, or it's going to crave ice cream, it wants tomatoes or it's going to crave ketchup, it wants potato or it's going to crave french fries, it wants minerals or it's going to eat dirt.

Chapter Endnote
The pyrex glass food containers that I keep referring to, come in four bowl sizes and three rectangle sizes. Here are their sizes.
1. Extra Small Bowl = 1cup 236mL
2. Small Bowl = 2cups 470mL
3. Medium Bowl = 1qt 4cups 950mL
4. Large Bowl = 1.75qts 7cups 1.65L 1650mL
1. Small Rectangle = 3cups 750mL (7x5x1.5 inches)
2. Medium Rectangle = 6cups 1.5L (8x6x2 inches)
3. Large Rectangle = 2.75qts 2.6L (9⅜x7¼x2¾ inches)
You'll need several of each size to make meals for yourself.

CHAPTER 43

What Works

As I write this, the news of the day is, "Science teacher loses 39 lbs in 90 days and 56 lbs in 6 months eating nothing but McDonald's."

The book, *The McDonald's Diet*, shows how teenagers, not experts, not doctors, not television personalities, proved the secret to fat loss. And so now you know. It's calorie control. This is why the Number Crunch Diet™ is the only diet I will ever use. I control the numbers, I control my size.

So this science teacher had his students choose his daily food intake strictly from the McDonald's menu. The total calories were 2000, and he also walked 45 minutes per day.

Walking is key to fat loss, and here's why. First off, you have to move your arms as you walk, opposite arm to leg, like cross-country skiing. Really picture in your mind the movement of cross-country skiing. Reach forward with your right arm, bringing it up high so that you can jab the ski pole into the snow ahead of you. Now, bring your left leg forward with the biggest stride you can make and then push your left leg behind you so that you propel your body forward. This is how you should be walking to lose fat. Why? Because this large opposite-arm-to-leg movement RE-CALIBRATES your hormones.

WALKING RECALIBRATES YOUR HORMONES™

NCD Recalibration Exercise™

This is why walking works. It's not that it's a great calorie burner, as there are better ways to burn more calories, but this opposite-arm-to-leg large stride large arm-swing action CENTERS YOUR BODY'S INTERNALS AND RESETS, RECALIBRATES, YOUR BRAIN, and hence, the hormones that your brain controls.

Get on a treadmill and set the speed to 4.0 mph, and walk. That is a pretty fast walk speed. You will need a large stride to keep up with the treadmill belt. Now, move those arms like you are cross-country skiing. Try it for one full minute. Then five minutes. Then twenty minutes. You will find that this takes concentration. You may experience your body wanting to tip to one side or the other as you walk. Keep working on this until you can consistently walk 15-20 or even 30-45 minutes perfectly.

You won't hear about recalibrating your brain and hormones on television, and people will put this idea down, but the naysayers are almost always the people who have never tried it themselves. Try it for yourself and see. Start with 3.5 mph or 3.2 mph if you need to. Just aim for smooth, uniform, large opposite-arm-to-leg strides.

So the science teacher lost about 3 lbs per week in the first 13 weeks, 90 days. His calorie requirement was likely to be about 3000 per day, as he's about six-feet tall with an active job and he walked 45 minutes a day. I would estimate that one-third of his weight loss was from water and gastrointestinal contents, and two-thirds was from body fat. So, 13 lbs of water and GI contents and 26 lbs of fat. That would be two pounds of fat loss per week. One pound of fat loss is 3500 calories, so two pounds is 7000 calories. If he needed 3000 calories a day to maintain, and he ate 2000 calories per day, he is cutting 1000 calories per day, or 7000 per week. So that's how he lost 2 lbs of fat per week, times 13 weeks equals 26 lbs of fat, and then 13 lbs of water and GI contents, comes to 39 lbs in 13 weeks.

Don't you love math!

GI contents. Hm. Never heard anyone refer to this before. They say, "Oh yeah, some of that was water weight." But I've got news for you people who are sportin' a belly, your gastrointestinal tract is backed up, and that backed-up GI tract is heavy.

Elvis Presley's colon upon autopsy weighed about 40 lbs. As did John Wayne's colon. The colon should weigh about 5 lbs. That means that these celebrities were carrying 35 lbs of backed-up GI contents. So when they say "water weight", we all know what's really happening. When you eat less, your stomach shrinks, and the excess GI contents leaves your body. Disgusting is right. This alone should motivate you to get to your ideal weight and stay there. And this book and the NCD Recipes™ can help you do just that.

So the science teacher and his students were successful at achieving fat loss through calorie control, i.e., number control, and walking to get the body moving and burning some calories with a concomitant recalibration of your internal mechanisms.

This diet also achieved another principle of the NCD and that is, getting it out of your system. He certainly got fries and a big-mac out of his system. But then again, maybe not. That flavor and those tastes may have an even deeper hold on him than they did before the diet. I can personally attest to the addictive qualities of McDonald's food, the chocolate shake is scary addictive. If you have one of those shakes, something in you wants more and more and more and you keep going back and back and back, to the pusher for more drugs. So when I read that food manufacturers and fastfood outlets put addictive chemicals in their food to keep you coming back, I knew instantly that this was true. I suspected it. My Internal Intelligence already knew it.

What else did this diet include? Well, mister science teacher started his day with a large diet coke for breakfast. This is cheating, and a NCD rule breaker. We already know the ingredients in pepsi, coke is essentially the same, but diet coke is worse, as now you're adding artificial sweetener to your bloodstream, brain, and endocrine system.

The NCD rules also include the following. You cannot make improvements if you continue to do bad things. In other words, no amount of good can compensate for the bad. Yes, people eat fastfood and then take a vitamin mineral supplement to compensate for a nutrient-deficient diet, but there are other nutrients they are not getting besides vitamins and minerals. The NCD only allows OCCASIONAL bad. Not daily bad, and not moderate bad. The recipes are 80-90-100% comprised of good nutritious food, with only 10 or 20% at the most of less ideal foods. But no obvious chemicals, and that includes artificial sweeteners.

Caffeine can be used strategically while you are cutting your calories. By strategically, I mean, on an occasional basis in very small amounts to carry you to your next meal if you find yourself on empty. This can happen, and when it does, I use three small squares of 85% cacao dark chocolate, made by Green & Black's. You can find them at Walmart for $2.97, but not all Walmarts carry them. Because they are organic, your healthfood store probably sells them, but the price may be higher. The bars are 100g 3.5oz and have 30 small squares. Crunching the numbers, 30 goes into 100g 3.3 times, so each square is 3.3g and 3 squares is 10 grams, or $1/10^{th}$ of the bar. If you had to resort to this back-up energy source once a day, then it would take you ten days to eat the entire bar. This is a conservative approach to theobromine/caffeine use.

Basically what I do is have one square in the evening if I find I want something but it's too close to bedtime to eat. Then after I have one square, if I want a second square, fine, no problem. Then if I still want one more square, then go ahead. The 3 squares 10 grams is equal to 63 total calories, and contains 15 calories of carbs, so this is not going to keep me awake when I go to bed. You can use this as a way to carry you to your next meal and to bedtime if you are cutting your calories. If you are on maintenance calories, you don't need caffeine. You have all the calories you need to get you through your day, providing that your calories are coming from macro-balanced Number Crunched Meals.

The NCD also uses this G&B 85% dark chocolate as part of the fat component in a few of its recipes. So for you chocolate lovers out there, you will enjoy a couple of squares for dessert, but not feel guilty because the calories are built into the meal.

If you would rather have coffee for those emergency energy situations, you could brew a pot of strong coffee or buy a 16oz cup of coffee at the AM/PM minimart which is usually strong coffee. Transfer the coffee to a glass bottle and place it in the refrigerator. Sobe beverage bottles are still made from glass and they come with a leakproof screw cap. As a side note, any time you see a glass bottle that fits your needs, buy it, take the label off and use it. These glass bottles are often worth more than the product they contain. As with the Sobe beverage bottles, I bought a case of 12 at S&F and poured the carrot orange drink down the drain, scrubbed off the labels, and kept the bottles. Perfect!

Take 1oz of your strong coffee and add it to 3oz of whole milk, and sip on it slowly, small half-ounce sips. This will allow you to have eight sips and it can carry you to your next meal. Those short narrow white- and red-striped straws work great for small sipping. The next time you are at a restaurant, ask your waiter to bring you a few of these straws from the bar. Then take them home. You can rinse them and reuse them. Or you can buy a big bag at S&F. In addition to making you sip slowly, they also keep coffee, or red wine, from making contact with your pearly white teeth!

Better yet, skip the caffeine altogether and use Nescafé decaffeinated coffee. Your milk drink will look the same and taste the same and your body will think it's getting coffee. Decaf does contain 0.3% caffeine, so it will give you a slight caffeine boost, but only if you're not a caffeine drinker. If you're a caffeine drinker you may have to use real coffee for a while before you can fool your body with decaffeinated.

This is why the NCD uses caffeine only as needed, in small amounts, strategically. Otherwise, you just keep needing more and more to get a boost from it. The point to remember is that caffeine is a drug, so treat it like a drug.™

The 3oz of whole milk is about 56 calories. Whole milk is the lowest in carbohydrate of all the milks, (nonfat, 1%, 2%, and 4%), so the sugars should be burned off before you go to bed. If you are experiencing low blood sugar from cutting calories, then you need this sugar. In this case, the NCD doesn't count these calories. It's only 56 calories, or 63 calories if you had the ten grams of dark chocolate, and since you are cutting 250 or 500 calories a day, then you still come in under at the end of the day. If you find you are having to fall back on this energy boost every day, then it's time to reevaluate your calorie cutting.

Avoid soft drinks for your source of caffeine because of the chemicals. HFCS is used in all major-brand soft drinks and is a chemical compound not found in nature, whereas the 85% cacao chocolate is organic and lists actual foods for ingredients, and coffee comes from a plant. Just remember, caffeine is energy without the calories. Whenever you get something for nothing, that's cheating. Use it wisely, and only when cutting calories.

If you worked out exceptionally hard and are having post-workout crash, use the ABC Water™.

Do not use caffeine to get you through your day. Eat according to the NCD and you should have all the energy you need.

So our science teacher is now famous for his diet that worked. Or at least in the short term. What is going-on on the inside? What about his food cravings for Teriyaki Chicken or Deviled Eggs, or simple apples and oranges and bananas? Oranges are another food I need on a regular basis. But it can't be freshly squeezed orange juice. It has to be orange juice from concentrate, with some of the pulp and orange peel. My Divine Intelligence made it clear to me that the freshly squeezed orange juice was missing some of what it wanted. So I went from spending $4.99 for a half-gallon of freshly squeezed orange juice, to spending $2.09 for a half-gallon of orange juice concentrate. These are very different products.

I also know that if I go more than 3-4 weeks without eating bananas, then one day when I walk into a supermarket and see those nice bright-yellow bananas, I buy eight and eat four that day and four the next.   So what's in a banana that my Divine Intelligence needs? I don't know, that's not my department, I just answer to it.

For the bodybuilder who wants fuller muscles, you can do the NCD One Fruit Meal™ instead of the FFS or HFFS as a way to keep your muscles fueled with carbs. I do this. If you work out and require 3000 calories per day, then have 5 meals of 40% carbs 30% fat and 30% protein, and one 500-calorie fruit 'meal'.

07:00	Breakfast	40 30 30 500cal
10:00	Shake	40 30 30 500cal
13:00	Lunch	40 30 30 500cal
16:00	FRUIT	500carbcals - bananas (5 small, 4 med, 3 Lg)
16:30-17:15		work out
18:00	Dinner	40 30 30 500cal
20:00	Meal	40 30 30 500cal

Your macros are 50% carbs, 25% fat, 25% protein. 3000x25% =750 calories of protein ÷4 equals 188 grams of protein, so about one gram per pound of body weight, the standard protein rule.

Science is years away from discovering all the intricacies. In the meantime, we all need to be giving our bodies what they require, and be doing so on a regular consistent basis, so that our desires don't turn into cravings, and so that our cravings don't morph into weird eating habits, like deep fat fried fake potatoes and black bubbly drinks with unnatural sugars and chemicals.

It will be interesting to see what mister science teacher will look like in twelve months, or, now that the diet is officially over, what he is currently eating. My guess is, he'll gain some of his weight back as there's no getting around your body's requirement for nutrients. The diet principle, the old calories in calories out, worked, but his food choices, well, even the dietitian sitting next to him said that she would have liked to have seen him eat 2000 calories a day from better foods.

CHAPTER 44

G LOAD

G stands for Glycemic, Load refers to the entire meal. Put them together and you have Glycemic Load, or, the sugar power of your meal, or, the insulin-spiking ability of what you're eating.

This is the most important word in your glossary of dietary terms. So take the words HDL and Cholesterol and move them to the bottom of your list and place GLYCEMIC LOAD at the top.

We have already discussed that the Atkins approach to fat loss is very effective because you cut carbs to a minimum and eat a lot of profats. Examples would be, a steak, protein and fat, or an egg, protein and fat, or dark meat chicken, or halibut, salmon, any time you eat protein and fat with no, or little carbs, the word "profat" is used. Nuts and seeds are mainly fat versus profat, as most nuts and seeds are 75-90% fat, with ~10% protein and ~10% carbohydrate. Exceptions being peanuts, 17% protein, and cashews, 20% carbs.

So, Atkins works because carbs are low, and sugar is low, and therefore insulin is low.

Insulin is the Master Hormone.™

Put that to memory. Insulin is the master hormone in your body. By master, I mean, it's the boss of the house. If insulin ain't happy, none of your other hormones are happy. If insulin is out of whack, all of your other hormones will be out of whack. If insulin is up down round and round, like a ride on a rollercoaster, so too will be your thyroid, your thymus, your adrenals, your brain, and your entire body's endocrine system. And this makes complete sense when you think about how important blood glucose levels are, glucose being your body's primary operating fuel.

So we need to control sugar consumption to control insulin levels to avoid diabetes and a whole host of other diet-related diseases, as well as to create a happy hormonal environment within the body.

We heard a lot about Glycemic Index several years ago, but the word has partially faded away, only to beat the drum louder and louder about cholesterol, HDL, and LDL. Move those to the bottom of your list. They are merely distracting you from the important indicators, Glycemic Load and Insulin.

Think of glycemic load as the glycemic index of your entire meal. Glycemic index is the sugar power or insulin-spiking power of a single food. Potatoes are high on the glycemic index because starch is just long chains of sugar. Nuts are low glycemic because they are low in sugar and the sugar is wrapped up in oil, fiber, and a little protein. When you wrap up the sugar, you lower its power.

Therefore, when you eat sugar with protein, you slow down the speed with which it enters the bloodstream and its insulin-spiking ability drops. When you eat sugar with fat, you slow down its insulin-spiking power, BUT, foods that contain carbohydrates and fats are foods like ice cream, boston-cream pie, cheesecake, and carrot cake. These desserts are dangerous to the waistline because, although the sugar is slowed down from 100 miles per hour to 60 miles per hour, it can still do damage and raise insulin. Then, as previously discussed, insulin comes along and takes the sugar and stores it in your body AND takes the fat from the cheesecake and stores it as well. This is why desserts are so fattening. CarbFats are a common dietary error because people fail to see the numbers.

CarbFats are allowed and are a part of the NCD plan, but only as incorporated into a meal, with sufficient protein.

In the diet book I just finished reading, the author, well-known, his recipes and recommendations consisted of a lot of carbfat meals. Sadly, he doesn't realize this and he's leading people down a wrong path. Carbfat meals look good on the surface, but numerically, they're a disaster.

You've got to crunch the numbers to see what you are really eating.

Another popular fat-loss author claims he's now figured out the real cause of weight gain and it's not calories, it's sugar. Again, leading thousands of his followers down a wrong path. I sometimes wonder if women buy into these male authors because of their good looks rather than for the value of what they are saying. Sugar is a factor, but it's not the big picture. Glycemic Load, Total Meal Carbs and Total Meal Sugar, is, and you certainly don't abandon the Total Meal Calories number either.

Let's look at the NCD Roast Beef Sandwich™ recipe. The recipe divides up, aliquots, into ten meals, each meal is 500 calories consisting of 40% carbs 30% fat and 30% protein. You could have two meals a day and finish the meals in five days. Typically when I make a recipe, I eat one of the meals as soon as I am finished preparing it. So, in this case, I eat one, and have nine meals remaining. Then if I eat another meal in three hours, I have eight meals remaining, and so two per day works out to just four days when considering expiration time, two meals on day zero, then two two two two equals four more days.

The NCD Roast Beef Sandwich™ meal consists of two slices of organic whole-wheat sprouted berry bread, 4oz raw 2.5oz cooked sirloin roast beef, and organic yellow mustard. For a vegetable, we add two pounds of organic carrots, either peeled and cut baby carrots, or full-sized carrots that you wash and cut but don't peel, and add these to the roasting pan. One-tenth of 2 lbs means you'll have about 3.2oz of carrots with each meal. Lastly, for dessert, we have 1/4th of a 73% dark chocolate almond bar with 15g of organic black raisins. Is this a party or what! I never get bored of eating these recipe meals. And more importantly, I never go away hungry or wishing that I didn't have to eat this boring salad with no dressing again. When I sit down to have a NCD meal, it's a party! And I party five times a day! I invite you to party along with me. In fact, I think the whole world should join my party!

Now let's examine the Glycemic LOAD of this meal. Where are the carbs and sugars? Two slices of sprouted berry bread, yes, 120 calories of carbs, but 16 of those calories are fiber carbs. Fiber is bulk, it's not used to produce energy, so we can subtract the fiber carbs from the 120, leaving us with 104 net carbs. Next, the roast beef. No carbs there. It's a lean roast that's 34% fat and 66% protein. Next, carrots, yes, 33 calories of carbs, but 9 calories of fiber, so 24 net calories of carbs. The dark chocolate almond bar, 3 squares 25g, 42 calories of carbs, 12 calories of fiber, 30 net carbs. And finally, the 15 grams of organic black raisins, jumbo raisins, by Sunview Farms, they are so big and plump, they are the only raisins I buy, and black plant food is like blackberries and bing cherries and the skin of an eggplant, full of rich color pigment, they contribute 47 calories of carbs, 3 being fiber, so 44 net calories from carbs. When we add up the total NET carbs of our meal, we have $104 + 24 + 30 + 44 = 202$. AMAZING! This is the foundational premise behind the Number Crunch Diet. Our meal is 500 calories, it contains 202 calories of net carbs, so 202 divided by 500 is 0.404 times 100 equals 40%. This is our 40% carbs.

Review the above example to get that down solid, because we are going to crunch some serious numbers in the recipes. Once you've got it down, then it's just repetition. So no worries. You'll be an expert at number crunching by the time you're done, and then you can design your own number crunch meals!

So how much glucose punch does this meal have? It's hard to say because no one's sent it off to a lab to have it analyzed. But, having had this meal many times, I can tell you it's just right. There is some sugar in the raisins and carrots that's available for digestion and to prevent the brain from getting sleepy, and there is some starch in the bread that supplies a gradual glucose release, and the whole thing is wrapped up in a mixture of protein, fat, and fiber, to further slow down the glycemic load. So my insulin spike is essentially zip, nada, zero. I haven't had my blood analyzed at 1-hour and 2-hours and 3-hours after this meal, but I can listen to my body's signals and tell. The more you can listen to and get in touch with your internal body, the less you will feel the need to rely on diagnostic testing and lab results. You will just know what's going on in your body, you will just know if your body is reacting to high sugar or not.

Internal people operate differently than external people. Internal people look to their Divinity to guide them. External people turn to the outside world, man and his technologies, to guide them. Making wise choices in life requires developing a communication line between the external you and the internal you.

So the next time somebody asks you, "What's your cholesterol, how's your cholesterol-HDL ratio, mine's 2.8 brag brag brag." Tell them, "I pay attention to more important parameters." Should they want to know your secret, do point them to where they can purchase this book.

Another factor influencing Glycemic Load is the speed with which you eat a meal. Eating and drinking is a lot like being transfused. The nurse hangs a bag of TPN, total parental nutrition, and infuses it over X number of minutes. If she pushes it in fast, the patient could react, if she gives it slowly, there's less likely to be a reaction. Certain of the NCD Recipes™ do contain some sugar. But we need sugar to supply our immediate needs, the needs of the digestive system, and the needs of the brain, which can require between 25 and 60% of the available blood glucose at any given time. We've all experienced that feeling of lethargy after a big Thanksgiving meal. All of our body's energy is going to our digestive system, leaving the muscles and brain short on energy and feeling zapped. This is why I stick with eating several meals a day, and only occasionally have a double meal of 1000 calories, and very rarely do I eat 1250 or 1500 calories at one sitting.

The NCD Thanksgiving Dinner™ takes a complete Thanksgiving dinner and breaks it into three separate meal recipes. It's awesome. While other people are moaning about how they feel, I'm zoom zoom. Holiday dinners are wonderful, but they can become predictable over the years. Try my healthier less calorie-burdened versions in *12 Changes A Year*, the companion guide to the NCD.

So back to our infusion rate. If we eat the high sugar meal slowly, we avoid an insulin spike. So, with the NCD Roast Beef Sandwich™ meal, the sandwich and carrots are eaten in about 15 minutes, and then the chocolate almond bar with raisins is nibbled on gradually for dessert, while you talk, or read, or you can take it "to go" and finish it at your desk.

In science, when you do a titration, you slowly add a solution to a beaker. Infusion rate, speed, titration, think of these words when you have a meal with sugar in it, and you can slow down that sugar by eating it over 30-45 minutes, a 30-45 minute infusion.

However, there are times when I need some sugar and I need it now. If I just came-in from doing yardwork or if I got home late from an appointment and I'm over my four-hour rule for meal frequency, then in these cases, I do gulp down half my NCD Flaxseed Shake™ immediately to get some calories into my body quickly.

Sugar has a function, to keep your brain and immediate body needs working. So use it, but use it as needed. The last thing you want is for your body to go into "Famished Mode" from withholding food for too long, and then you eat everything in sight and of the wrong things. This is where a high-glycemic shake can halt that need for calories and prevent famished mode from occurring. If you work out at the gym or take a boot-camp class or do sweat cardio on a treadmill, and you don't eat a meal within one hour after the class, then two hours later your body goes into Famished Mode, and then you eat 1200 calories in 20 minutes. Not good. So use sugar wisely and understand what affects its speed, power, and punch, understand the principles of Glycemic Load.

CHAPTER 45

THE RECIPES

I hope you are starting to get the feel for the Number Crunch Diet, its principles, its rules, the justification for them, and the recipe structures. You will prepare the recipes, make X number of meals, and you're good-to-go, fuel and nutrition, to live and work and do.

The main obstacle is likely to be time. Cost is not that much because you have to buy food regardless, and the money you will be saving on eating out will allow you to afford good-quality groceries. And, just like you need tools in the garage, you need tools in the kitchen. Spend your money where it counts, where it will pay off for you in the long run. And use your free time wisely, take your lunch break alone and review a recipe, then make a list and plan a strategy for making it. Two years from now people will be asking you what you are doing, while they go over to pour themselves a coffee and take a cookie from the table. Be a role model. I know you've got it in you to be the best you can be. Be that best! You've only got one chance at life. Go For It!

Now you may think, I will just throw a little of this together with a little of that and divide it up and that's close enough. Sorry, it's not. The NCD recipes came to me as Divine Revelations, flashes of insight, and each one of them is no different than walking through an art gallery. Many of them came to me perfect on the first go-around. Some were perfected the second time around. Others I played with to make more of the meal from scratch, and so it evolved. Neil Sedaka said in his live performance, "These songs are like my children." That's kind of how it feels with the recipes, each one being a unique creation, some better than others, but all contribute to the overall repertoire of the Concert Of Meals.

So start by following the recipes, then when it becomes ingrained in you, you can spread your wings and try designing your own recipes. Or, if you send me your requests, I'll see what I can come up with. My recipes reflect meals that I like to eat and may not, in fact guaranteed to not, cover all people all cultures all tastes.

Also, the food items used in the recipes are purchased at my local supermarkets. If you happen to live in California, well, good for you as you will recognize their names. But clearly, I cannot find food products for each reader living in a different part of the country. You will have to shop around and try to find a close match. For example, the NCD Hawaiian Pizza™ calls for two 20oz cans of chunk pineapple. That's easy, as all the brands are pretty much the same. Pick one that just says "Pineapple and Pineapple Juice" as you don't need citric acid to maintain freshness if they canned it properly. However, the recipe calls for three 6oz packs of Trader Joe's Canadian-Style Bacon. This is a key flavor ingredient, along with the TJs Fat-Free Spaghetti Sauce. I have purchased Canadian-Style Bacon at Albertson's Supermarket but it's not the same. The hogs were raised on different feed. Hence, the pizza will be good or very good, but it won't be amazing. The important part is to find products that match the percent carbs, fat, and protein, so that your meals come out 40 30 30 and 500 calories. So do the best you can to purchase the brands that are used in the recipes, or, do the best you can to find a close match from the stores where you live.

Additionally, the NCD recipes result in virtually no leftover or partial packages. For the NCD Hawaiian Pizza™, you need five different food items and eight total items, you use all eight items in the recipe, and when you are done, you have zero leftovers and six personal pizzas, each consisting of 500 calories with 40% carbs 30% fat 30% protein.

Hot out of the oven, I typically eat a double meal, 1000 calories, and then one more later in the day. Then two the next day and one the day after that. If you can buy the exact ingredients and prepare it exactly as instructed, you will never have a better Hawaiian Pizza. It's one of my best recipes and one of the first I ever designed.

So this is why the recipes make 6 meals or 8 meals or 14 meals, because you use everything that the recipe calls for so that there are no partial packages when you're done.

Now, if the recipe calls for eight ounces of pepper-jack cheese, you can certainly buy the 8oz size and have no leftovers, or you can buy a larger size to save money. I used to buy just the 8oz size because I didn't want to deal with leftover partial packages, but now I buy the 5 lb size of pepper-jack cheese at Smart & Final. I use 8oz for the recipe and vacuum seal the remainder. This is something you can do as you grow with the recipes, but first just make them as is, then if you want to tweak the recipe to save money, by all means go-for-it.

Here's the recipe I made yesterday, the NCD Chicken Bowl™. Add a 2 lb package of brown rice to a glass bowl, add water and microwave it for 15 minutes, it's "parboiled" so it's quick-cook rice. Then, boil 5.3 lbs of chicken breast. Slice and dice it when it's done. To an extra-large bowl, add six cans of organic pinto beans, the brown rice, and the diced chicken breast. Mix and aliquot it into 21 medium pyrex bowls with the red lids. To serve, I take a 12oz container of pico-de-gallo and add 4oz to my chicken bowl. Then I add 86g of guacamole, about 3 weight ounces, and voila, Pollo Bowl, as good as any place I've eaten it. I tried to save money by using dried pinto beans, but the canned pinto beans have perfect texture and they don't cost that much plus they're organic. I tried to make my own pico-de-gallo or use a giant can of a different brand but it didn't have the zing and so I didn't enjoy it as much. You might be thinking 21 servings are way too many. Well, this recipe is one of the few that is this many, and I'm okay with it because it's so delicious and nutritionally satisfying that I eat three meals the first day and then three meals pretty much every day for the next week. Plus, now I don't have to cook as much, so if I have work to do I can get it done without being interrupted with meal making. The top shelf of my freezerless refrigerator has 21, or 18 remaining, meals ready to supply all of my energy needs. Plus I have other meals on shelves two and three, so I'm stocked fueled and productive. I'll make this recipe again in 12 weeks, 4x a year.

By the end of the week, my 21 chicken bowls are gone, and so is my desire for rice beans salsa and guacamole. Guacamole is another one of those foods my Divine Intelligence asks for on a semi-regular basis. And I can't go more than two weeks without eating chicken or my DI will be asking for that too. I can also tell you that as long as I am eating beef, I will have no desire for a fastfood burger. If you have urges for a fastfood burger, your body is simply wanting beef. Make it yourself, the NCD Double Cheeseburger™ or the NCD Bacon Cheese Burger™, and you won't have any cravings for fastfood versions.

Guys who work out can easily consume 3000-4000 calories or more a day, so 21 meals can be used up in 5-6 days in these cases.

If you are cooking for a family, these 21 meals are enough for dinner, plus breakfast, lunch, and snacks for everyone for the next 24-48 hours.

Another nice feature of the NCD recipes is the price per serving information. Most of the meals cost less-than $3. The NCD Chicken Bowl™ meals are $2.93 each, so half the price you would pay at a fastfood outlet, plus you're getting organic rice and organic pinto beans, and real guacamole, not the kind they squirt from a gun, and not a tiny dab either. When I made the pico-de-gallo from scratch and used dried pinto beans, I was able to bring the price down to $1.67 per meal. Pico-de-gallo is ridiculously overpriced, but they know that very few people have the time to chop up tomatoes onions cilantro and jalapeño peppers on top of preparing the rice beans and chicken. The NCD recipes are a mixture of good-quality packaged foods and food from scratch.

If you eat five NCD meals per day at $3 apiece, that's $15 a day, or $450 per month for high-quality homemade meals.

It's this high-quality homemade nutrient-dense food that will make your food cravings fade away. With the NCD Chicken Bowls, when I have finished the 21 meals, I've had 4 lbs of guacamole. That's some serious healthy omega-9 dietary fat. Plus all of the other nutrients contained in the other ingredients.

Here is another key point, and that is, don't be caught without meals. Every day spend a little time preparing food. It may just be prepping food for the next day when you will make a recipe. Or, if the meal has two parts, make one part today and the other part tomorrow. Just get into the habit of spending 10-15 minutes minimum in the kitchen each day. Open your refrigerator and ask yourself, "What can I prep in advance?" I often boil the chicken breast the day before, and then the next day, it's just a matter of assembling everything and dividing it up.

With practice, you will be able to pump those meals out in record time. I can make six Hawaiian pizzas in 35 minutes, with all the dishes washed and everything cleaned up and put away. Dividing 35 by 6 and you end up with about six minutes of food-prep time per pizza. You have time for that.

I really believe that the overweight problem is really a nutritional-deficiency problem for many people. The NCD requires that you make your own meals, with the recipes to assist you. Eating out is no way to get good nutrition, and the hidden calories and hidden food additives won't get you to where you want to be. Had mister science teacher assigned his students to pick foods from a supermarket, instead of from fastfood, and had them create a recipe repertoire during his six months of dieting, then his students would have really gotten something from the course that they could take with them for the rest of their lives.

Chapter Endnote: Pico de gallo, a kind of salsa, is really spelled as three words, no offense to the hablan español grammarians!

CHAPTER 46

WHOLE GRAINS

The Number Crunch Diet is against whole grains. This is just more dumb advice coming from the so-called experts being interviewed on TV. Never once have I heard these people mention

SPROUTED GRAINS

Sprouted Grains have been on the shelves of supermarkets for the past ten years and still all we hear of is whole grains. What people think are whole grains are processed grains. The only true whole grains are things like Wasa Crackers, the ingredients say, "whole grain rye flour, salt" that's it. Two ingredients. No conditioners, no stabilizers, no words you can't pronounce. Ryvita is another company that makes whole grain crackers, and there are a few others. For bread, only purchase sprouted bread. The grains are partially sprouted to create a more living food product. Just like how you would grow alfalfa sprouts in a sprouting jar, creating live living plant food, so too is the sprouted grain bread.

So forget about Whole Grains right here right now. Grains are what bulk up animals, so you're just adding bulk to an already bulky body. Are you starting to get the picture that you and the mass public are 50-60-70-80% misinformed? Not everything in the media is misinformation, but you have to analyze it for truth. Don't just buy into whatever they are telling or selling you. Be alert and aware and awake. Save the autopilot mode for the beach, but the rest of the time, you need to be alert and discerning.

You may think, "Whole grain rye flour and salt, that's a pretty dull cracker." Wrong wrong wrong. Top that cracker with some sliced turkey breast, sliced cheddar, and sliced dill pickle, and boom!, you have the NCD Crackers Turkey Cheese™ meal. I love this meal, and because it's low in carbs, you get to have for dessert, a Bartlett Pear. Yes, I meant for that to be anticlimactic. You don't need a mocha chocha chocolate blah blah blah. You need nutrition. And to make your calories count. Think about your internals. And feed that. I make this recipe every fall when pears are in season and look so good. But you can't just go and eat a whole pile of pears or you'll gain weight from all the sugar. The NCD recipes allow you to have 200 calories of carbs with every meal. If you have five meals a day, that's 1000 calories of carbs per day, 200x5.

The key is that you have to pick and choose your carbs. Don't just eat carbs out of habit. And don't eat carbs that you don't particularly want. And you can't have double carbs, i.e., a roll and potatoes. It's either a roll OR potatoes. Nor can you have triple carbs, a roll, potatoes, and a glass of wine. And quadruple carbs with the sherbet dessert, well, I'm not even going to address that.

Think about the amount of empty calories in one hamburger combo meal. Top and bottom bun, or some burgers come with a middle bun as well, deep-fried potato starch with sugar ketchup, washed down with a 100%-sugar fountain drink.

If this is you, repent from your ways and move forward to taking control of your health and becoming a new, healthier, more productive you. Fast food is Fat food. And dead, nutritionally. The deep-fried oil in the fat fryer ought to turn you away from french fries forever.

Say, "Today! I commit! to transitioning from a fastfood diet to that of making my own meals!" "One year from today I WILL be well on my way! to achieving this goal!"
Signature:_____   Date:_____

In the 1970s they used to use lard in those deep fryers. Then they switched to corn oil, and then to "healthier" canola oil in the 1990s. Some places boast that they fry in peanut oil. It really doesn't matter what oil they use because the temperature is 425 degrees and so if they started out with fresh oil in the morning, by lunchtime the oil is BURNT and by the end of the day it's BLACK. And most eateries don't change the oil every day. That would be way too costly for them. If you happen to be the first customer on the morning that they change the oil, well, lucky you. Deep-fried food is poison, don't eat it. Your body doesn't have any use for oil that has been heated to 425 degrees. In fact, it's the exact opposite. Your body has to take that burnt oil in your meal and detoxify it and eliminate it. Eating deep-fried food is one of the BADs that no amount of GOOD can correct. You simply must put an end to this bad dietary behavior. There are better ways to cook your foods than by submerging them in boiling hot oil.

To satisfy the need for french fries, the NCD has two recipes, NCD Salmon & Steak Fries™ and NCD Pork Chop Mushroom Gravy Steak Fries™.   Ore-Ida fries in the freezer section of your supermarket are fine to eat every so often. The label reads, potato, vegetable oil, that's the not great part, and then it lists a "pyrophosphate", which literally would mean a phosphate molecule on fire, attached to a sodium. Probably not what your nervous system needs, but occasionally is fine. You can also, cut up potatoes, steam them to soften them, and then bake them in the oven with some coconut oil or butter. The mushroom gravy or ketchup is what gives them the flavor anyway.

Keep in mind that if you eat potatoes, such as baked potato with sour cream and scallions, or meatloaf and red potatoes, you won't have any desire for the weird versions. The closer you can eat to the original form, the less you will want of the adulterated forms.

Eat the real thing and the craving for the processed thing will fade away.™

So forget about whole grains. You can have true hearty whole grain crackers, or sprouted grain bread.

Now the NCD does allow you to eat what you want, so there are times when I want a crusty roll or sourdough loaf, or even garlic cheese-toast with plain-white french bread, the NCD has you covered. There are meals for all of these, you make them, eat them, and get it out of your system.

Generally though, for the past several years, I haven't had any desire for french bread, even when it's staring me in the face at the checkout stand. I just look at it and see it for what it is. Empty over-processed nutrient-depleted calories. I don't shop with my eyes anymore, I shop with my internals.

The point of this chapter is, you don't just eat bread thinking that, "I need to get my X number of servings of grains per day." Nor do you look at bread and think that it's acceptable food. It's fun food. All carbs are fun food. You're allowed 200 calories per meal of this fun food so pick and choose them wisely.

The reason people are carrying around excess fat is because the media keeps telling people to eat whole grains. News Flash! There Are No Whole Grains! Food Maxx has zero whole-grain bread products on their shelves. And it's the same for most supermarkets. You have to go to an offbeat supermarket like Trader Joe's or the healthfood store to find true whole grains, or sprouted grains. And the media know this. They know that, "If we can convince the public to keep eating grains then we can keep billions of dollars coming in for our fat-loss industry." The fat-loss industry is no different than the medical industry. They partially help you, but then they partially let you fail, so that they can fully keep your money.

JUST SAY NO TO WHOLE GRAINS.™

The carb and fat portions of your meal are the party parts. Remember, carbfats are "dessert" foods. You can have them, but only a portion. So ask yourself, "What do I want for carbs?" Then have exactly that. Up to a 200 calorie limit per meal, four or five or six times a day. If you eat 2500 calories a day, then you are allowed 1000 calories of carbs per day. That's a pretty good party. And don't forget, you can do it all again the next day too. 1000 calories of carbs is 250 grams, this is TEN times the amount of carbs that you would eat in the initial weeks of the Atkins diet. If you can do Atkins, you can do the Number Crunch Diet.

Now, if you want to go full desserts, full carbfats, then you add to your 200 calories of carbs 150 calories of fat, like the carrot cake example. But, like the carrot cake example, you also have to include 150 calories of protein, the skillet chicken. Now, I don't suggest that you go full desserts all the time, but, the point is, and this is key, you can eat these foods, these desserts, and not get fat because the dessert is the carbfat portion of the meal.

No other diet that I am aware of does this.

When it comes to whole grains, sadly, the media has done such a mind-job on most people that when I explain to someone that your choice for carbs should be from plants and fruit, and that whole grains are really nutrient-depleted processed grains, they look at me like there's something wrong with me. They give me that look like, "You probably think that the fluoride they put in the water is bad too." Yes, I do.

Read the book *The Fluoride Deception* by Christopher Bryson and then I'll be happy to discuss the subject matter with you. If you should come up against someone who challenges you on urine pH or addictive chemicals in the food or whole grains, just ask them what book they are basing their information on. They will likely say, "I heard it on the news" or "That's what everyone believes." Well that's why everyone's in trouble. Why do you think they call it Television Programming? You know, years ago when television first came on the scene, many parents wouldn't let their children watch it because they felt that the TV programs were…programming their children. Those were some very astute parents.

Whole grains is simply an agenda to make and keep you fat.™ And then what happens when you become overweight? What? Oh yeah, you go to see your doctor. Hm. Funny how that works.

Chapter Endnotes
Just so you know, "pyro" has to do with how much water is contained within the molecule.

backup
back up
back-up
Wouldn't you like to know the difference in these three words? Of course you would!
The first is the noun form, "This is a nice backup."
The second is the verb phrase, "It is backed up."
And the third is the adjective form, "The backed-up GI tract is..."
You'll be an expert at math and English by the time you're done!

CHAPTER 47

REVIEW

So let's review. The NCD™ is a calorie counting diet whereby you count meals and snacks. The recipes are Pre-Counted™ so that you can keep track of your daily and weekly total calories easily. A meal is defined as 500 calories and a snack is defined as 250 calories. A snack can be an actual snack, such as the NCD Franks & Fruit™ which consists of two jumbo beef franks with mustard and 75 calories of fruit for dessert, totaling 250 calories, 40% carbs 30% fat 30% protein, or it could be half a meal.

Although the meals are "500 calories", that does mean plus or minus 5-10%, so 475-525, or 450-550. The NCD Southwest Steak Bowl™ is 543 calories with 63 calories of fiber, half your RDA of fiber in each meal! So 543 minus 63 is 480 net calories. Please understand that I am using the Nutrition Facts on the product labels and they are not always that accurate. In certain situations, I may go a little higher or lower depending on how the meal feels. If the meal feels a bit heavy, I may increase the carbs a little to 42 or 44%. The steak bowl is made from four foods, and when it divides up the numbers are 42% carbs 28% fat and 30% protein. When the macros are calculated using the net carbs, with the fiber calories subtracted, they become 35% carbs 32% fat and 33% protein. The meals are targeted at 40 30 30 and 500 calories, with reasonable variability.

We already know that if you control your calorie intake that you can lose fat, as proven by the science students who controlled their teacher's diet. Weight Loss or Weight Gain or Weight Maintenance is a Numbers Game.™ Primarily.

We already know that extremes in macro percents is a radical approach and that your body's homeostatic mechanisms want to keep things the same, so a moderate approach is more likely to fool your body into shedding pounds without it noticing.

We also know that low fat, high fat, low carb, high carb, is again, going from one end of the spectrum to the other end, and that the NCD a third a third a third approach is more balanced, since you need all three foods, carbs fats and proteins, as they all play important functions in the body. Plus, food tastes better, and meals digest better, and nutrients absorbs better, when you have some of all three foods present at each meal.

Additionally, because you are not limiting carbs or fats, you get to include all possible food choices in your diet, no exclusions.

EXCEPT, chemicals and poisons. Ingredients listed on the label that you don't recognize as foods, just assume it's an additive. I buy my cottage cheese at Trader Joe's because the brands at Food Maxx and Walmart have additives. The Sunny Select brand plain 2% cottage cheese has "Natural Flavor", which is what? What? When you see the ingredient "natural flavor" the NCD says what? It's a code word for "Chemical Additives That Make You Addicted To The Food." So, French's Mustard company, if you are reading this, stop hiding behind words that the consumer cannot understand. Be like your competitor Heinz and list all real foods on your ingredients label. The NCD is a chemical additive free diet, allowed rarely or occasionally only.

High-fructose corn syrup is poison, as is hydrogenated or partially-hydrogenated oil, aka, margarine. As is deep-fried food cooked in burnt cheap oils found in most restaurants and fastfood outlets. And, I am not even going to discuss olestra, fake fat, and artificial sweeteners, fake sugars. If you can't see that these are chemicals, well, I can't help you. You've lost your ability to see the obvious.

The Number Crunch Diet is a way of eating whereby you make your own meals, as nutrition and number control are key principles of the program, eating foods that your Divine Internal Intelligence needs to run its body.

Notice I said, "its" body. Your body doesn't belong to you. It belongs to your inner you, your Inner Divine. The Higher part of you. The Holy part of you. Connect with that and you'll be able to see right foods from wrong foods.

The meal frequency of the NCD is often, every 2 or 3 or 4 hours, and avoids going 5 and 6 hours without eating. In my particular case, I eat all day. If your goal is to add muscle and gain weight, and you are working out hard 3-5 times a week, you likely need 3500 or 4000 calories a day. This means eating every two hours, 7 to 8 meals a day. I've done this calorie intake before and you literally feel like you are eating all day. Just keep that freezerless refrigerator stocked up with breakfasts, lunches, dinners, and shake meals, work out, eat, recover, sleep, and GROW! Your diet makes or breaks your progress.

As previously discussed, the macro percents can be modified in either direction to achieve your desired results. If you want more fat loss, then drop the carbs to 35% and raise the fats to 35% while keeping the protein at 30%. If you want still more fat loss, drop the carbs to 30%, raise the fat to 40%, and the protein 30%. This is moving you towards the low-carb diet, but not radical. If you want to gain weight and have a fuller-body look, drop the fat to 25% and increase the carbs to 45%, keeping the protein at 30%. This can easily be done by eating 40 30 30 MTWRFSa, and doing Fat-Free Sunday, where you eat 2000 calories of fruit, spread out throughout the day, plus two chicken breasts, or scrambled egg whites with tabasco or ketchup, or fat-free ham and fat-free turkey slices. The 2000 calories of fruit carbs will reload your muscles with glycogen for the following week. If you want to drop your percent fat to 20, then eat 40 30 30 MTWFSa and do FF Thursday and FF Sunday.

First, you need to get control of your calorie intake, utilizing the NCD recipes, and then once you have control and you know your daily requirements, then you can adjust the macros, if you want to. It is easy to lose weight or gain weight by eating 40 30 30 seven days a week, just cut out a snack or meal, 250 or 500 calories, from your day, or if you want to gain weight, just add an additional snack or meal to your day. It is not necessary to modify the macro percents. In fact, the 40 30 30 fuel formulation provides a stable nice steady supply of energy. It's low moody, and no rollercoaster.

Again as previously stated, the recipes are made using foods found at my local supermarkets. You will have to search for similar products in your area. Full details of each food item are provided, including the nutrition facts, container size, and ingredients, so this should help you to find a similar product. Pay attention to ingredients. In addition to "natural flavor" being in the cottage cheese, I also saw some brands that had "titanium dioxide" as an ingredient. Titanium dioxide is used in soap to make it white. Titanium is a metal that they use to coat drill bits to make them five-times stronger than steel. You can also find titanium in golf clubs and titanium dioxide used in sun reflectants on the roofs of buildings. The makers of certain cottage cheese brands think that this is okay to put in your food. What do you think?

So, your strategy is to buy the exact or similar food items, prepare the recipe according to the directions, then aliquot it into the number of servings given in the recipe, keeping your refrigerator stocked with homemade meals to fuel your energy needs.

If you start with one recipe and make it twice in one month, then move to another recipe the next month, then 12 months from now you will have 12 recipes in your recipe repertoire. Do this again the following year and your repertoire will consist of 24 recipes. At that point, you are fully qualified to Number Crunch Design your own recipes. Congratulations in advance! You're a graduate of the Number Crunch Diet!

CHAPTER 48

Customizing

Now, the NCD can be adapted to people who are responsible for making meals for the whole family. The Hawaiian Pizza is easy, as the recipe divides into six individual pizzas, you can double or triple the recipe depending on the size of your family. If there is someone else in the family that is battling with their weight, you can teach them the principles of the NCD, and have them follow what you are doing. The meals are very balanced and satisfying. The macros and the calories are so ideal that you may notice that people don't eat as much. They will sense that feeling of, "I'm done, that's enough" and stop eating naturally. Too much carbfat and you don't get that satiated feeling that protein gives you, and too much profat doesn't provide you with enough carb energy for digestion.

So when the recipe says to divide it into 12 medium pyrex bowls of 450 grams each, you can weigh out 450g onto a plate for yourself, and eat at the table with your family. Everyone's food portions at the table are different, men typically eat larger portions than women. Your 500-calorie meal won't look as big as your husband's, but it won't look small either. So you won't feel embarrassed by the size of your meal. It will look appropriate and normal. In fact, a year from now, mom might be looked at as the only one in the household with sensible eating habits.

The other thing you can do is, when the recipe says to aliquot it into 12 medium pyrex bowls of 450g each, you weigh out 450g into each of two bowls and put them in the refrigerator for your breakfast and lunch tomorrow. This way you have your meals, 500 calories and 40 30 30, available and ready for you to eat when the time comes. In other words, after you make a recipe, pull 2 or 3 or 4 aliquots off for yourself, and let your family have the remainder. If you need a snack, 250 calories, later in the evening, have half of one of the meals.

If someone says, "Let's have lunch at XYZ restaurant tomorrow." Say to them, "Let's meet at the park, I'll bring two meals, and we can have a PICNIC." This is so much fun! At first people are a little hesitant, but then the kid in them says, "Yeah! why don't we do that!" You save a bunch of money, you eat healthier food, you're outdoors, and who knows what other beautiful event might occur. A squirrel may come to visit, a blue jay may drop by, you get to see people playing, exercising, and just having good old-fashioned outdoor fun. In the summertime, the most popular tables at a restaurant are the ones on the patio. In 2012, the Earth Day holiday theme was "Go Outside And Have A Picnic". Take your two medium pyrex bowls of NCD Four-Bean Chicken Salad™, a tablecloth, some cutlery, and your ABC Water, and your friend will think you are the coolest person. You'll both go away smiling.

So any time the recipe says to aliquot it into a certain-sized glass container, either the pyrex type or the SKS glass jar with screw cap type, you are always free to serve it directly onto a plate. All of the recipes will tell you how many grams you need in order to have a 500-calorie serving. So it doesn't matter too much what container, or plate, you divide it in or on to, as long as your servings are X number of grams. Just keep in mind that the SKS jars with screw caps extend the expiration of your meals by double and triple because of their airtight seal.

Get used to using your scale and measuring amounts in grams, or in weight ounces. It's faster and more accurate than measuring by volume using measuring cups and spoons, and fewer dishes to wash. The NCD Caesar Dressing™ requires seven ingredients, and if you use the EXACT amounts, you get the EXACT fantastic flavor each time. Too much or too little lemon juice, or too much or too little garlic, and the recipe doesn't come out the same and the flavor is not quite right.

So measure your food and ingredients in grams and weight ounces using the S&F scale, the 10 lb capacity one, and count your energy intake in calories. DO NOT count your intake in grams, such as, "I had 50 grams of fat today." This is just another way to make you lost and confused and ultimately fail. Counting in "points" is worse. There are no textbooks that refer to the energy of metabolism as "points". Diet plans that use this are just adding their own layer of confusion on top of an already confused populace. Energy is measured in calories. Check with your high school biology or physics teacher if you don't believe me.

The NCD plan measures food by WEIGHT, (grams or ounces), and tracks energy intake in CALORIES.

MEASURE by WEIGHT

Track your ENERGY intake in CALORIES

This is science, food science. I am not inventing some crazy tracking and measuring system. For those of you that have "points" ingrained in your brain, please click on "delete" and "yes". Very Good.

The conversion from grams to calories is:

Carb grams times 4 = calories
Protein grams times 4 = calories
Fat grams times 9 = calories

So, 4 4 9. When it comes time for you to Number Crunch Design your own recipes, that's what you will use. But the NCD recipes are already number crunched so you don't have to. During your first year of building your recipe repertoire, try to play around with the numbers and master the conversion and percent calculations until it becomes mindlessly easy for you (and it will). Then the next time you're at the mall standing in front of a display that says "30% off all items" you will blurt out the cost of the item in seconds and your kids or spouse or girlfriend will look at you like you're some kind of mathematical genius. When that happens, don't gloat, or you'll blow it, just stand there, humbly knowing that you've earned it.

Another feature of the NCD is that it's a bit raw. I am a big believer in eating 80% of your food raw and 20% cooked. When meat is cooked, like chicken breast, it's cooked to MW, medium well, that means there is just a slight bit of pink on the inside. Then you remove it from the heat and allow it to cook OFF HEAT to well done. This way you are cooking it just enough, without overcooking it and killing your precious proteins. Same for beef, which I prefer MR, medium rare. You cook it to rare, remove it from the grill, and then allow it to finish cooking off heat to MR. Perfect. Cooking your meats to just the right doneness is crucial, not only for taste and enjoyment, but most importantly for the proteins. If you like your beef done medium, then remove it from the grill when it's MR and it will continue to cook off heat to medium. Just don't overcook your proteins.

Overcooking the protein is so typical of many restaurants. You might as well not even eat the meat or fish as it's not going to do you any good. I paid a hefty price for a lobster dinner at a well-known chain restaurant and it was cooked to death and salted beyond repair. This, and many other experiences, tells me that when people are cooking, they are not thinking about the amino acid molecules and proteins contained within the meat. In fact, most restaurants are so concerned with bacteria that they are extending the cooking times just to be safe. Well, the bacteria are dead, but so too is the protein. Those of you who buy protein powder know that the label is supposed to say "Undenatured", meaning that the processing was done at low temperatures to protect the amino acids and proteins from structural damage. Heat-damaged proteins don't function well within the body.

I got my first job at a steakhouse in the late 1970s and about once a week someone would order a steak "Blue Rare". This means that you just place the steak on the grill, flip it, turn it, flip it, to create the waffle pattern, and off it goes to the customer. The steak is raw. One time, a customer didn't even want it on the grill at all, but the law required having to put it on the grill, but it didn't specify for how long. This particular customer wanted to eat it raw right from the refrigerator. The NCD isn't that raw. It's 80/20. An emphasis on raw, but not crazy raw. Although, I've never eaten a blue-rare steak, so it may be that these blue-rare customers know something. What if we really aren't supposed to cook meats and proteins?

Abnormal protein shapes are seen as "foreign invaders" by your immune system. So, not only does your Divine Intelligence not have the right-shaped protein to use, your immune system is going on the attack after the wrong-shaped protein. This is why the NCD Off-Heat Cooking™ method is so important. If you do it just right, then your Divine Intelligence is happy and your Immune System is happy. If you eat overcooked proteins, it's a double negative. You fail to nourish your body with useable protein, while simultaneously flooding your bloodstream with denatured proteins that your immune system has to eliminate.

Could food allergies, autoimmune disease, colon disorders, all be rooted in overcooked denatured abnormally-shaped proteins?

The same is true for overcooked oils. Those 425 degree oils. They're dead. Unusable. Or worse, the burnt oils get used. The body decides, "Well, if burnt fat is all I have to work with, then I'll just have to make a cell membrane from burnt fat." You're in big long-term trouble if your cell membranes are being made with burnt oils and hydrogenated man-made fats.

Contrast that with fats from nuts and seeds, avocados, olive oil, high-quality dairy, and high-quality lean meats, fish and poultry.

Which category are you in? The NCD will get you on the right path. It's as much about Education as it is about Number Control.

The NCD Off-Heat Cooking™ principle applies to vegetables as well. Cook your broccoli three-quarters of the way, and then allow it to finish cooking off heat. I used to blanch my broccoli and green beans to give them that nice green color. Blanching is where you take the vegetables out of the boiling water and then submerge them for a few seconds in cold water to stop the cooking process. Unfortunately, your vegetables turn cold by the time you sit down to eat them. Those fancy culinary schools will likely switch from teaching blanching to their students to teaching NCD Off-Heat Cooking™ once they read this book. Now, instead of blanching, I create that same bright green color by removing it from the water when it's ¾ done. Then it finishes cooking off heat, and the vegetables are still hot when you sit down to eat them.

Optimum nutrition is best obtained by paying close attention to your cook times and aiming to cook all foods exactly right. This is the "love" component of a homemade meal, because someone was watching over it and pulled it off the heat at just the right moment. The NCD recipes provide detailed instructions including how many minutes of cook time to use to help you avoid overcooking your nutrients, rendering them void, or worse, harmful. We want delicious, not deleterious. With regard to customizing, just be certain to make the recipe as instructed so that it comes out 40% carbs 30% fat 30% protein, and then serve yourself a 500-calorie portion by weight.

Chapter Endnote
Coming up you are going to see, Omega 9 6 3. In numerical order, it's 3 6 9. But when referring to their double-bonds, it's 9 6 3.
Omega-9 = 1 double bond
Omega-6 = 2 double bonds
Omega-3 = 3 double bonds

And just to fill in the rest:
Saturated fat (animal and coconut) = no double bonds
EPA = 5 double bonds
DHA = 6 double bonds
You'll get it at the end, :)

CHAPTER 49

OMEGA 3

One of the unique features of the Number Crunch Diet is the NCD Flaxseed Shake™. There are three versions of it so I never get bored. But first, let me clarify what an Omega-3 Fat is, because the way the current terminology is being used is confusing.

The way I see it, we have five kinds of edible fat.
1. omega-9 = monounsaturated fat = olives/oil, avocados, peanuts
2. omega-6 = polyunsaturated fat = corn, safflower, sunflower oils
3. omega-3 = polyunsaturated fat = flax, chia, and hemp seeds
4. omega-3 = DHA and EPA = salmon, mackerel, sardines, fish oil
5. saturated fat = animal and dairy fat, also plant coconut oil

So, immediately you should see that #2 and #3 are both being called polyunsaturated fat. This is terrible terminology because omega-3 from flaxseed is essential and we need more of it in our diets, and omega-6 from refined corn and safflower oil is junk oil.

They are planning to revise the Nutrition Facts label and sadly this clumping of good omega-3 in with bad omega-6 and calling them both "polyunsaturated" is not helping the consumer at all. If I had not studied this in depth, I would definitely be confused about fats.

So, forget the word "polyunsaturated" fat.

While you're at it, forget the word "monounsaturated fat" as well.

These terms are too general, preventing you from seeing clearly.

Call olive oil, avocados, and peanuts, Omega-9s, corn, safflower, and sunflower oil, Omega-6s, and flax seeds, chia seeds, and hemp seeds, Omega-3s.

Now the next thing you should have noticed that's not right, is that they are calling fish oil omega-3. Stop calling fish oil omega-3 fat. Instead, refer to it as fish oil or DHA and EPA.

So our new, NCD Fat Definitions™, are:
1. Omega-9
2. Omega-6
3. Omega-3
4. Fish Oil
5. Saturated

Animal, Fish, and 3 6 9 Plants. Put that to memory.

Land and Sea fats, and three plant fats.

These are the 5 Edible Fats. Notice I said edible. Margarine is not edible. Cut a stick of butter in half and then rinse the knife with water. The butter comes off completely. Cut a stick of margarine in half. The margarine sticks to the knife. When you rinse the knife with water, it doesn't come completely off. It leaves a greasy gluey film. Picture this gluey lipid in your bloodstream. Not good.

Along with hydrogenated and partially-hydrogenated fats being unedible, so too are deep fried fats in that deep fat fryer people like so much. These two fats are toxic health-damaging fats. The NCD says NO to both of these, not even rarely or occasionally, so cross them off your list and as of this day forward you refuse to eat them, and this includes indirect forms, as when used in packaged foods.

NCD NonEdible Fats™
~~Deep Fryer Burnt Oil Fat~~ – not edible
~~Hydrogenated Man Made Fat~~ – not edible

The next fats that you are going to say NO to are the Omega-6 fats. If you've paid any attention to the health warnings over the past several years you will have heard that we are eating WAY too much omega-6 fat and not enough omega-3s. Some reports say we are consuming as much as 15-20 times too much omega-6. And let's face it, corn oil and safflower oil and cottonseed oil and sunflower oil are just inexpensive low-quality oils. So scratch Omega-6 oils off your list.

NCD No Omega-6 Oils™
~~corn~~
~~safflower~~
~~cottonseed~~
~~sunflower~~

Sunflower seeds and corn on the cob or frozen or canned corn are good and fine, and a few of the NCD recipes have corn.

NCD Corn & Sunflower™ rule
The foods are fine, the refined oils are not, too high in omega-6 fat.

Soybean oil is not a good choice for oil as it is likely from genetically-modified soybeans, unless you purchase organic soybean oil from the healthfood store. The NCD says rare to occasional only, with regard to soybean oil.

NCD Soybean Oil™ rule
Organic or Nonorganic, rare to occasionally only is okay, when part of another food as listed on the ingredients label. No liquid soybean oil that you buy and use for cooking, baking, or salad dressings. Its 50% omega-6 fat content and high probability of being GMO make this not a good choice.

NCD Canola Oil™ rule
Organic canola oil is fine for sautéed and stir-fried meals as it's light and tasteless so it will take on the flavor of the dish. But cook in water and add the oil OFF Heat to protect the oil. Like soybean oil, canola is not a great oil, so only occasionally, and buy organic

from the healthfood store. Organic means no GMO, but most importantly it means no SOLVENTS used during the extraction process. You don't want to be eating trace amounts of paint thinner with your oil. Look for the words "No Hexane" on the label.

NCD Stir-Frying & Sautéing™ rule
Rather than stir-frying or sautéing in oil, do it in water, then remove the pan from the heat and add some garlic-infused organic canola oil and toss. Let the cooking process finish Off Heat with the oil being protected. "Stir-Frying" can be accomplished by boiling vegetables in water to ¾ doneness, drain through a colander, let drip some, then place the vegetables in a large container with lid, add the oil, close the lid and shake. Much healthier and it tastes the same, better actually.

The Asian way of stir-frying food in hot oil, is the same as the Western way of submerging food in deep-fryer oil. They're both bad and outdated cooking methods that damage your health.™

NCD Boiling Preference™ rule
Recall how water is an absorber, it draws things out, it's a dissolver. Rather than submerge your food in oil, submerge it in water. Boil it. Boiling-water pulls out fat from the chicken making your chicken leaner. And, water pulls out impurities and any remaining pesticide residues that weren't removed during the washing of your vegetables. Boiling also cleans any spoiled areas that weren't cut out, maybe you didn't see them, and it pulls those spoiled areas out from the food and into the water. Just be sure to remove your chicken from the water at MW doneness, and remove your vegetables from the water at ¾ doneness, allowing them to finish cooking to "just right" off heat. Plus, the maximum temperature reached during water boiling of your chicken protein is 100°C or 212°F. This is half the temperature of deep-frying and stir-frying.

Boiling cleanses, purifies, and detoxifies your vegetables.™

Boiling is less damaging to meat proteins and removes fat.™

NCD Olive Oil™ rule
Use olive oil Uncooked. It has a low burn point, so its place in the diet is in homemade mayonnaise and salad dressings. This is a good source of omega-9 nonessential fat. However, you may not need much olive oil if you are eating omega-9 from peanuts and avocados. If you don't eat peanuts, peanut butter, and avocados, guacamole, then yes, you should be consuming olive oil. The point being, you don't need all three forms of omega-9 each week, just pick one per week.

For baking, use coconut oil as your first choice and butter as your second choice. Both are saturated fats and are heat stable up to 350 degrees. The preferred choice is coconut oil since we get enough dairy products already and the NCD Popcorn™ and the NCD Curry Chicken™ both use butter. Therefore, in order to get coconut oil in our diet, use it in baking. It is also used in the NCD Skillet Potatoes™, which gives them a fun coconut flavor. Although both of these fats are Saturated Fats, one is an animal product, containing a small amount of cholesterol, and the other is a plant product with zero cholesterol.

NCD Skillet Greasing™ rule
For skillet greasing, use coconut oil or butter, or organic canola or coconut spray is also acceptable. But read the label. Coconut spray has "natural flavoring" in it. My coconut oil nonstick spray is interesting. It is from organic coconut oil, because the ingredient says "organic extra virgin coconut oil", but there is no "USDA Organic" logo on the product. Nor does it say "Organic" on the front label. So what's going on? It's organic but it's not labeled as organic. The product is indeed organic, however, the company decided not to pay the extra money to become government certified. These organic farmers have been farming organically for decades. Organic is all they know. Organic crops are all they've ever grown. So there's a trend among organic farmers to save the consumer money by bypassing the cost for government certification, which apparently is quite expensive. This additional cost gets passed on to the consumer. This trend by these organic farmers is allowing for prices to be reduced by 10-30%.

One summer while traveling through British Columbia Canada, I stopped at a roadside fruit stand to buy some cherries. Wow. They looked beautiful, but they had a faint white film on them. I ask if this was from pesticides. Well, she looked at me like I had just offended her and said with her eyes "you stupid Americans". She informed me that, they don't use pesticides, none of the farmers use pesticides, and that faint white film was due to the high calcium content of the artesian water used to wash them. Oops. My bad. Apparently pesticides, and all the other "cides" are an American thing. Small countries don't use pesticides and everything they grow, feed to their livestock, and eat for themselves, is organic.

So since my nonstick organic coconut oil spray came from Sri Lanka, but it doesn't say "USDA Organic", but the ingredient says "Organic", I'm okay with that if it saves me money. This is also the only coconut oil spray that I've seen that doesn't have "Natural Flavoring" as an ingredient. So I like the fact that these Sri Lanka farmers aren't into chemicals period. It has just two ingredients, the organic virgin coconut oil, and the non-chlorofluorocarbon propellant. Oh yeah, the old sprays used to contain chlorofluorocarbons that would break down the protective ozone layer surrounding the planet. Oh boy.

Clearly there are two types of food manufacturing, Good and Evil.

So our NCD Edible Fats becomes:
1. Omega-9 = olives, avocados, peanuts
2. Omega-3 = flax, chia, hemp
3. fish fat
4. animal fats and coconut oil

Nuts are a mixture of 3, 6, and 9, and even some saturated fat. The NCD recipes include nuts because nuts are good for us, but we don't concern ourselves with their oil composition because they are a mixture. There is one nut that is higher in omega-3 than all the other nuts, and that is, walnuts. In fact, Diamond Corporation, the maker of nuts in the baking aisle, was sued for claiming that their walnuts contained omega-3. But it's true. Walnuts are 5th on the list, tied with wheat germ, for omega-3 fatty acid content. But we live in a world where you can't make a claim, not even a true scientifically-documented claim like walnuts being a good source of omega-3, unless the government says so. So apparently, if science says it's true, it's not true until government says so. I think this is what people are referring to as big government.

Why don't they put a warning label on colas that the phosphoric acid leaches calcium from your body, and that, if consumed long term could result in needing a hip replacement or dentures?™

The NCD recipes will have you eating nuts instead of cereals for breakfast.   Brazil nuts, cashews, hazelnuts, pecans, almonds, walnuts, macadamia nuts, whatever nuts you like. I am not a big fan of pine nuts, but if you want them, you can substitute them in, or design a recipe with pine nuts. I'm also not a big fan of sunflower seeds, pumpkin seeds, or pistachios, but if you like them feel free to use them instead of cashews in the recipe. The nut portion of the meal is made more appealing by adding a small amount of chocolate, chocolate sauce, or other surprises!

It's better to get your nuts with a little chocolate, than not at all.™

The NCD Favorite Breakfast™ includes one slice of toast with peanut butter and jam or banana, and this is how you will get omega-9 fat and get that desire for peanuts out of your system. So for your omega-9 sources, rotate, NCD Favorite Breakfast, peanuts, with NCD Chicken Caesar Salad, olive oil, with the NCD Chicken Bowl, guacamole. Pick one a week. Your body can make omega-9, so don't think of it as Essential. Needed for nutrition yes, but not essential.

The essential fats are Omega-3 Flax, and fish oil DHA and EPA. Omega-6 is technically essential because we cannot make it, but we get plenty already, so we don't need to go looking for them. The two dietary fats that most people are low on, and that we need to actively "Seek" are, Omega-3 and Fish Oil.

NCD Dietary Fats Explained™
1. Omega-9 = we can make this, plus we get it by eating OAP
2. ~~Omega-6~~ = we can't make it, but we don't need more
3. Omega-3 = we can't make it, and WE NEED IT
4. DHA EPA = we can make some, and WE NEED THEM
5. Saturated = we can make it and we need it, but we get plenty

DHA and EPA are special fats, because they function like hormones. Good Hormones. Our bodies can make a small amount of DHA and EPA from omega-3, but the conversion rate is small, only 2.7 %. But the good news is, if we are consuming omega-3 fat, then we can make DHA and EPA. These two special fats are also found concentrated in the adrenal glands, testes, brain, and retinas. So if you want these organs to work right, you will want to be consuming fish oil DHA and EPA, and foods that contain them.

There are three other oils that have hormone-like effects, because they contain a high percentage of GLA, gamma linolenic acid.
1. Borage Oil 20%
2. Black Current Seed Oil 15%
3. Evening Primrose Oil 9%
GLA gets converted to PG1, prostaglandin series 1, which reduces water retention, thereby reducing blood pressure, it has anti-inflammatory effects, calming arthritis, PMS, and other inflammatory conditions, and it blocks a pathway that produces PG2, prostaglandin series 2, the bad guy. Your body can make GLA, but if it's not making enough of it to keep up with your condition, you may find that supplementing with Borage Oil may help. I've never supplemented with these but I am considering purchasing borage oil for flare-ups, as the science on this is solid.

So our goal is to get Omega-3 fat from flax, and DHA and EPA from fish, since most of us don't eat enough flax, chia, and hemp, we are deficient in omega-3, and because most of us don't eat enough fatty fish, we are deficient in DHA and EPA. We need to "seek these out" and start eating them regularly. Similar to our alkaline reserves, our omega-3 and fish oil reserves are low and we need to get them stocked up and then keep them stocked up.

There are also eight essential amino acids that our bodies cannot make, and all of the vitamins are essential by definition, we cannot make them. Plus all minerals are essential.

ESSENTIAL means you must CONSUME them.

NCD Dietary Essentials™
1. sugar – none
2. plant fat – omega-3 flax
3. fish fat "hormones" – DHA EPA
4. 8 amino acids – ILLM PTTV
       Isoleucine Leucine Lysine Methionine
       Phenylalanine Threonine Tryptophan Valine
5. all vitamins
6. all minerals
7. all phytonutrients, color pigments found primarily in plants

Do you see how a bad diet of, fastfood, processed food, refined food, overcooked denatured food, man-made adulterated food, is going to be missing a lot of the Essentials? Add to that the BAD things found in junk food and deep-fried food, not only are you not getting enough GOOD, but you are flooding your system with BAD. Bad food choices.

Part of the blame falls on our culture. Our ancestors, who lived off the farm, and other cultures around the world who don't live in cities, they don't eat the way we do. Walk into any cafeteria and the majority of the people are ordering cooked eye-tantalizing food without any awareness of why they need to eat in the first place.

The food our ancestors ate, food that was close to its origins, is quite different from what most of us are eating today. Is it any wonder that Americans consume 50% of the world's prescription drugs and 80% of the world's painkillers. I think our diets and lifestyles play a big part in this. What do you think?

Health problems are due to a decades-long lack of Essential Dietary Nutrients, in my opinion.™

The NCD has two recipes that include Canned Salmon, which is preferred over frozen salmon because the oil in the salmon is protected from light and therefore protected from oxidation. Fresh salmon is exposed to both light and air. You eat salmon for the oil, the DHA and EPA benefits, and those oils are very sensitive to oxidation by light and air. Canned salmon is protected from both.

The NCD uses canned salmon, instead of fresh or frozen salmon, for its air and light protective packaging.™

See, who out there is telling you that the oil in your salmon is being oxidized by light and air? But it's completely true. Read the book *Fats That Heal Fats That Kill* by Udo Erasmus, PhD. It's a 450-page action-packed book that took me four months to read. They started bottling olive oil in dark bottles to protect it from light, right? I wish they would stop packaging nuts in clear-plastic bags. Apparently they remove the air and replace it with nitrogen gas, which eliminates the oxidation caused by oxygen, but I would rather they just suck out the air by vacuum sealing and use opaque bags. Vacuum-sealed food contains almost zero air. Put vacuum-sealed food in the refrigerator and you extend the expiration by about ten times, depending on the food and how good of a vacuum and seal you were able to achieve.

If you haven't already done so, purchase a vacuum sealer. They are well worth the investment. I have the Food Saver Vac 300, and it's a workhorse, very reliable and well made.

Oils need to be fresh and protected from oxidation, not just from oxygen, but from light as well. In nature, nuts are grown in airtight light-protected shells. We rarely think of them in shells because most supermarket nuts have been removed from their shells. But nature grows them in shells for a reason, to protect them from air, and from light.

Have you ever walked into a fish market and it smelled of fish? Bad fish. Smelly fish. That's the fish oils gone rancid. This is why many people don't like to eat fish because most of us have eaten rancid fish, and now our body is saying "Yuck, stay away from fish." Fish has to be eaten immediately, or else freeze it or can it. 24-hours later and you're pushing it. 48-hours later and it's halfway spoiled. 72-hours later and it's completely spoiled. And if you let fish sit out in an open-air display, it's spoiled within six hours. Hence, the fish-market rancid-oil bad-fish smell.

The flax seeds that I purchase come in vacuum-sealed opaque bags, nice. The website is www.bcof.com Bush Creek Organic Foods. If you buy 12 one-pound bags of organic golden flax seeds it will cost you $84.35 with shipping, so that works out to $7.03 per bag, plus they throw in a free coffee grinder! They are some great people, and their website is very informative so go there and check it out. You might want to place your order now so that you're ready to make the NCD Flaxseed Shake™, and start supplying your body with regular fresh doses of the best-quality highest source of omega-3 on the planet.

NCD Fresh Oil™ rule
Unlike the other plant oils, omega-3 oil, once ground, is good for only 2-3 days in an airtight container, in the dark, in your refrigerator. The oil in fish is even more unstable. Fish must be consumed, frozen, or canned, the same day it is caught. Nuts, seeds, and other oils, do contain some omega-3 and so ideally these need to be eaten, vacuum sealed, or frozen soon after being opened from their shells.

Oils turn rancid by the oxidation from air and from light.™

Fish DHA and EPA oils turn rancid in one day. Flax seeds last indefinitely, but once ground they are stable only 2-3 days when stored properly. Their lack of stability stems from the "U" shape of their fatty acid chains. This "U" shape is unique to these fats, making these two food sources essential to our diets. Functionally, this unique "U" shape makes cell membranes flexible, giving them the ability to bend and contort as they move around and press up against other cells. This U-shape also opens the "doors" to the inside of the cell, allowing larger molecules to pass in and out.™

225

So I hope you can see that not all fats are the same. The bottom line is, that the good fats allow your body to operate properly, without problems, and to last a long long time, and bad fats do the exact opposite.

Jesus ate fresh fish and so did his disciples, but they didn't fry it in a deep fryer, although the Bible doesn't say this, I'm fairly certain they didn't. And just like the cranberry, flax seeds were made for a specific purpose in "mind".   The next time you look at the convoluted grooves in a walnut, ask yourself, "What part of my anatomy has this same convoluted appearance, and its round ball-like shell looks very familiar, hm?" Omega-3

Chapter Endnotes
Yes, yes, don't begin a sentence with a numeric, "24" "48", yes, I get that. And don't hyphenate before "later", I get that too. My apologies to all the grammarians reading this. "Grammarians", not sure if I would want to join that club anyway!

And for the record, the correct spelling is "inedible".

CHAPTER 50

PHYTONUTRIENTS

I've mentioned this word before and it simply means, color nutrients. Plant Pigments. The NCD is big on nutrition. Although you can eat whatever you want to get that food craving out of your system, once you have kicked the habit, you should naturally choose foods that are healthy and top-of-the-list is Phytonutrients, living plants with color pigments.

I bring attention to this because, like the Flaxseed component, the glycemic LOAD principle, and sprouted bread over whole-grain bread philosophy, the emphasis on getting living plants from the six color pigment groups, is foundational to the Number Crunch Diet™.

I track what plant colors I've eaten and if I see that I've gone without eating Red for more than two weeks, I choose my next recipe to have a red fruit or vegetable in it. Same thing for Yellow, Orange, White, Green, and the Purple-Blue-Black group. I also track my dietary intake of Leafy Greens, as these are special in that they are loaded with vitamin K and chlorophyll. Leafy greens help support the lungs, without which, we would cease to live.

So the seven categories of plants, six colors and one leafy green, are listed below. All are fresh unless where noted.

1. WHITE

Fruit Interior
apples – fall, winter
bananas – year round
pears – fall, winter
Vegetable Interior
cucumber – regular or English
mushrooms – fresh or canned
potatoes – STARCH vegetable
yellow or white onion – good source of sulfur
radishes – onion-like properties and DIM
turnips – DIM
garlic – good source of sulfur and antimicrobial properties

DIM stands for Di Indolyl Methane, die-in-doe-lill-methane, diindolylmethane, found in cruciferous vegetables. The four main ones are, Broccoli, Cauliflower, Brussels Sprouts, and Cabbage. Memorize these four. Radishes and Turnips are secondary in DIM content.

Why are these important? They lower estrogen. A lower estrogen level means that you have a relatively higher testosterone level. The world adores men exuding testosterone. Even in women. When a man's T level drops, so goes his "mojo". He loses his effectiveness to lead his family and perhaps his staff or downline. He's flat, flaccid. Women would do wisely to keep their estrogen levels under control as well by avoiding plastic water, pesticides, synthetic chemicals in cosmetics and medicines, and allowing their testosterone levels to be in charge of their temperament. Be a woman on the outside, but be a bit like a man on the inside. To help with this, the NCD recommends that you rotationally eat broccoli, cauliflower, brussel sprouts, and cabbage each week.

NCD Four T Vegetable™ protocol
week 1   steamed organic broccoli or ¾ boiled nonorganic broccoli
        with a 5g sprinkle of parmesan cheese
week 2   brussel sprouts ¾ the way boiled, cut in half, with 5g PC
week 3   cauliflower ¾ boiled with a sprinkle of parmesan cheese
week 4   NCD Coleslaw™

Any time you get a vegetable, pat yourself on the back. For this reason, many vegetables in the NCD are free. You don't count the calories. Four ounces of broccoli has 21 calories of carbs and 11 of that is fiber, so 10 net-carb calories, and 16 calories of protein. The 10 net-carb calories are so minor that you will likely use double that just to chew and digest it. A small sprinkle of parmesan cheese is also pretty minor, depending on your sprinkle. My sprinkle is typically about a half tablespoon, equal to 15 calories, 6 of which is protein. If I get lavish and have an entire level tablespoon, then it's 30 calories. Not a problem.

To get used to doing this, place the bowl of 4oz broccoli or brussel sprouts on your scale, press on, press grams, then shake parmesan cheese onto the vegetable until you have five grams.   This is 20 calories of parmesan cheese, still considered free since most people can burn off 20 calories in no time. The 4oz of broccoli with 20 calories of parmesan cheese is not what makes people fat.

Having a DIM vegetable with a 5g sprinkle of parmesan cheese is a great way to carry you to your next meal or to bedtime, if you are cutting calories and find yourself slightly hungry.

Bodybuilders, these are your four T vegetable snacks to support your testosterone level naturally with food.   BBCC, Broccoli Brusselsprouts Cauliflower Cabbage.

2. YELLOW
Solids
pineapple – fresh or canned
mango – seasonal, fall, spring
bell pepper
lemon
Exterior
plums
corn – STARCH vegetable
zucchini
dates – sugar
curry, turmeric, curcumin – spices

Dates are brown in color, but I don't have a brown category so I just put them here in Yellow. You are free to create your own list if you don't agree with mine. Or there may be fruits and vegetables that I am missing, figs for example, I'm not much a fig eater, although they are quite good if you buy them at the right time.

Note, be sure to buy mangoes when they are on sale at the front of the produce section, otherwise you will pay three times the price. I usually buy twelve mangoes when they are two-for-a-dollar or three-for-a-dollar and eat them on Fat Free Sunday and get them out of my system. This way, I am not paying $1.49 for one mango when they are out of season. Plus, when they are out of season at the higher price they don't taste as good. A ripe mango should look nice on the outside, and then "give" a little when you press it with your thumb. But if you buy them when they are on sale at the front, then you don't need to check for ripeness, as they are in season, perfect looking, and prefect ripeness. So watch the flyers that come in the mail, or check your local supermarkets online for their fresh-fruit specials, and be sure not to miss that one- or two-week window in the fall and usually in the spring.

The NCD Lemonade™ is like nothing you've heard of before, and it's so delicious, satisfying and nutritious. Lemons are your body cleansers, just like how they are added to cleaning products to create a clean fresh scent, they keep your body clean and fresh on the inside.

Yellow bell peppers are a great way to get a lot of yellow plant pigment without the sugar of pineapple or mangoes, or the starch in corn. Cut, cored, and sliced, you can eat them as a calorie-free snack, or mix them 50/50 with green bell peppers.

Of the nine Genetically-Modified Plant Foods grown in the USA, Alfalfa, Corn, Canola, Cotton, Papaya, Soy, Sugar beets, Squash, and Zucchini, ACCC PSSSZ, you can see that zucchini, yellow and green, are listed as GMO crops.

GMO is when they take DNA genetic material from one species

and splice it into the DNA of another species, cross-species genetic manipulation. Apparently, in order to keep up with the growing demand for salmon, scientists have engineered genetically modified fast growing giant salmon, which are photographed and stated as being four-times larger. Having seen wild salmon, I will say that they are bigger, but not four-times bigger. I would say they are about the same length as wild salmon, just fatter. So, they're more like genetically modified fast growing obese salmon. The government hasn't approved them, but if it does, it would be the first animal/fish GMO to be sold in supermarkets, as currently we just have the nine plants. Whenever it comes to something new, I usually wait. Let the other people try it first and I'll decide in ten years. This is new science and no one knows the long-term consequences of eating GMO foods.

I do understand that man is trying to feed the ever-growing population and conserve the wild sources, and GMO probably makes sense on paper. But the NCD is not a big believer in man-made foods, so as long as nature's food is still available, eat that.

So when you buy corn or yellow or green zucchini, buy organic to avoid GMOs. Or look for "Non-GMO" or "GMO-Free" on the label, which is the fastest-growing product label in history, so clearly, the public is unsure about consuming Frankenfoods, despite how "safe" they tell us it is.

The NCD Garlic Green Beans™ are tossed in organic canola oil with garlic, and stevia is used to add sweetness without carbs. Canola works good for this recipe as it has no flavor and so it takes on the flavor of the garlic, and it's lighter than olive oil, but since it is organic it's non-GMO. The calorie-free stevia sweetener comes from the leaves of the plant, and the NCD uses it only occasionally. Garlic, well we all know how good garlic and onions are at being anti-microbial, keeping viruses and bacteria at bay, but their sulfur content supplies your body with this essential mineral required for healthy skin, joints, and cartilage.

Don't forget that you can consume GMO corn, soy, and alfalfa indirectly by eating nonorganic livestock products. Grass-fed cattle and feedlot-fed cattle result in two different products, even though they appear to be the same. It's like margarine and butter. They look the same but molecularly, they are not.

I've never been a fan of papaya or squash so you won't see NCD recipes that include these. Nothing wrong with them, but just be sure to buy organic to avoid GMOs.

Soy is found in the soybean oil of the NCD Coleslaw™ dressing, so that falls under the rare-to-occasional rule.

Sugar beets are not to be confused with purple beets, which are listed in the purple-blue-black category. Sugar beets produce table sugar, so buy organic to avoid GMOs as it's about the same price, and if you see sugar as an ingredient on a food label instead of organic sugar, you can assume it's from GMO sugar beets.

The yellow pigment of curcumin, found in turmeric and curry spice, is an excellent antioxidant. All spices are antioxidants, but yellow curcumin is the champion. Buy three big shakers at Walmart for $2 each and fill one with turmeric, one with curry, and one with ground cloves. Buy whole cloves and grind them in your coffee grinder for a fresher better taste. Cloves aren't yellow but they're anti-parasitic. Begin sprinkling them on your meals, chicken, eggs, fish, and vegetable sides, just a little sprinkle is all you need. When we think of cloves, we think of ham, but try it with a fresh-baked fish fillet and melted cheddar.

3. ORANGE
Fruit
cantaloupe – late summer
cantaloupe juice – see below
oranges – winter
orange juice – from concentrate
tangerines – winter
tangerine juice – "Cutie" brand has 35 tangerines in a 48oz bottle
apricots – summer, or dried

peaches – summer, frozen or canned okay
nectarines – summer
Vegetables
carrots – preferably with the green tops on them
carrot juice – homemade or store bought
pumpkin – canned
sweet potatoes – STARCH vegetable
bell pepper

For the cantaloupe juice, wash your cantaloupe in hot water and remove any blemishes, hopefully there are none, if you do this in late August when they are in season and on sale, they will look perfect on the outside. Then juice the entire thing, seeds, rind, and flesh, for a fantastic-tasting nutrient-rich vision-support beverage. If you've never juiced an entire cantaloupe before, you've got to try this. Just be sure to do it when they are in season so the fruit is perfect looking on the outside and full of flavor on the inside.

For the bodybuilder, nothing beats the NCD Orange Shake™ for a complete dose of macronutrients, including whey, but from food, (not from powder), plus oranges and tangerine juice. The recipe makes nine, and I often finish them in 3-4 days and repeat the recipe midweek. The taste reminds me of the old Orange Julius drink or an orange creamsicle, but instead of artificial flavor, the Number Crunch Diet uses real foods for flavor.

Apricots, peaches, and nectarines, be sure to eat these when they are in season and get them out of your system until next summer. You don't want to be buying dried apricots or canned or frozen peaches during the off-season because you missed eating the real thing in July.

Carrots and carrot juice, my Divine Intelligence won't let me go more than a couple weeks to a month before it says, "Hey! I need carrots in here!"

What better way to get the benefits of pumpkin than from the NCD Pumpkin Shake™. Mmm! And sweet potatoes are another great way to get solid orange color, as in the starch component of the NCD Steak & Eggs™ recipe.

Get into the habit of eating all of the color categories of fruits and vegetables on a regular basis to avoid becoming

VEGETABLE RESISTANT ™

Vegetable Resistant is when you don't like to eat vegetables anymore, you've gotten out of the habit of eating them, and that's when you hear kids say, "I don't like vegetables," or you see adults picking a certain vegetable out of their food. Their taste buds have drifted off in the wrong direction.

Next up, RED!

Chapter Endnote
The T-vegetable group is a legitimate category, but just don't get the idea that they are "steroid" vegetables.
GMO labeling is under attack, just look for organic, or the "9" prefix on the produce code, i.e., 4011 is a banana, 94011 is organic.

CHAPTER 51

Phytonutrients Part 2

4. RED
Fruit
pomegranate – fall
pomegranate juice – store bought
watermelon – spring and summer
watermelon juice – see below
grapefruit – ruby red
grapefruit juice – store bought
cranberries – Thanksgiving & Christmas
California cherries – June July
raspberries – fresh or frozen
strawberries – spring summer, or frozen
goji berries – see below
the skin of red grapes, red raisins, and red wine
Vegetables
tomato – fresh, canned, sundried
bell pepper

Notice that there is really only one primary red vegetable source, tomatoes. My internal intelligence regularly wants tomato products, tomato sauce, cherry tomatoes, sliced vine-ripened tomatoes, diced canned tomatoes, sundried tomatoes. Tomatoes tomatoes tomatoes. Be sure you are getting them and you won't want the salty processed version, ketchup. Keep sundried tomatoes stocked in your fridge for a NCD free-vegetable snack of RED.

Buy pomegranates when they are in season in the fall and eat them on FFS, HFFS, One Fruit 'Meal', or as the fruit/dessert portion of a meal. Eat them and get them out of your system until they go on sale and are in season again next year. A pomegranate is a "superfood", so luckily we can purchase pomegranate juice year round. You will enjoy a 6.5oz serving per meal, times 8 meals, equals an entire 52oz bottle of pomegranate juice with the NCD breakfasts, so buy a Ninja Blender!

Watermelon, never miss a season of watermelon. They are loaded with red color, if you buy the seeded ones. Seedless watermelon, man-made hybridized watermelon plants engineered to produce fruit without seeds, is more pink than red. I hope you are getting me when I contrast God's way versus man's way. He's God with a big "G" for a reason. I do buy a seedless watermelon occasionally as it does have a different taste and texture, and the NCD rules do allow for occasionally of the less-ideal foods, but make God's versions your first choice, and man's versions an occasional treat.

Watermelon juice, similar procedure to the cantaloupe juice, wash in hot water, remove any blemishes, but also remove and discard 3/4ths of the rind, then juice the watermelon, seeds and all, with 1/4th of the rind. Use a fresh watermelon in season and you will be amazed at the freshness and flavor of this drink. Mmm!

Ruby-red grapefruit is another way to get some calories to carry you to your next meal or to bedtime if you are hungry for something. The NCD Grapefruit™ consists of taking a 5 lb bag of ruby-red grapefruits, peeling them all, and then aliquoting them into 3oz servings, the SKS 8oz glass jar with screw cap is perfect and allows for extended expiration, up to two weeks. I typically end up with 18 servings of 3oz each. Each serving is 33 calories of carbs with 4 calories of fiber, so 29 net-carb calories. The NCD puts the 3oz grapefruit serving in with the "Free Vegetable" category because grapefruit is good for you, any time you get one you get a pat on the back. There's a 6th way to nip a food craving in the bud and that is with "bitters". But not the one in the grocery aisle, the one in the alcohol aisle, and I'll explain this technique in the recipes. Grapefruit has a partial "bitter" effect, curbing your desire for food. But I keep a steady supply on hand in the refrigerator for Red, and for Citrus vitamin C. I miss them if I don't have a serving or two a day. It's that DI thing again, it talks, I listen. The 29 calories of carbs is not going to blow your numbers and make you fat. If you need a little something, then have a little something. But better that it be 3oz of grapefruit than a slice of toast with peanut butter and banana, carbfat, "dessert"! If you finished working out at the gym, have 3 servings of 3oz grapefruit as a muscle filler-upper. But be sure to wait about one hour until your next meal, because you just gave your bloodstream a mild sugar boost with 3 servings, equal to about one large grapefruit, or ~90 calories. Just remember to listen to what your body signals are saying. If you don't free hungry then don't eat and wait until your next meal. If you need a small, medium, or large boost, then have one, two, or three servings of the 3oz grapefruit.

Cranberries! Our special berries that are acid producing in the body instead of alkaline producing. I buy them in November and then again in December and make the NCD Cranberry Sauce™ and get my craving satisfied until next Thanksgiving. Once you switch to eating fresh cranberries in season, you won't go back to canned cranberries. They are two nutritionally different products.

California cherries are red and Washington Bing cherries are purple/black so they are in the PBB color group. Last year I was up by the San Francisco Bay area and I purchased some of the best cherries I've eaten in 30 years. Mmm! The bing cherries seem to be getting sweeter each year and I almost don't like them anymore because they taste too much like sugar and not enough like cherries. But these California cherries were Awesome!, full of that red cherry taste with just a normal amount of sugar.

Have you noticed the words "Super Sweet" on fruit packages? The bing cherries in the 2 lb plastic container had "Super Sweet" on the label. And a pineapple at Costco had "Super Sweet" on the paper tag. If you are reading this bing cherry and pineapple growers, we don't want SUPER SWEET candy fruit. We want fruit that has flavor. We want fruit that tastes like fruit, not like sugar. Now, I keep a watchful eye out for "Super Sweet" on the label and I don't buy it. It's hybridized. They're just creating more diabetics. Like what they did to the corn, they bred the fiber out and turned it into high glycemic corn.

Raspberries and Strawberries, get them while they are in season and on sale because as you are well aware of, blueberries, blackberries, raspberries, and strawberries are EXPENSIVE off season. Blueberries are like gold now, a 2 lb bag is nearly $10. I remember when a 1 lb bag of frozen blueberries was $1.29. Now it's a 12oz bag for $2.99. I've even seen a 6oz container of raspberries sell for $5.99. That's a dollar an ounce for fresh raspberries. So pay attention to that one-week window when they go on sale and get your fill of them so your body's stocked up with these nutrients until next year.

Goji Berries. This is new for me. I buy organic goji berry juice puree at www.bioinnovations.net along with their Noni juice and Acai. I encourage you to invest in a case of these and it's usually 50% off with free shipping, terrific savings. You won't find a better quality product anywhere. It doesn't taste that good because there's no sugar in it, but that's how it should be, no sugar. Have you noticed that we are a culture addicted to sugar? What is the statistic, 125 pounds of sugar per person per year? Or it keeps climbing, now it's 150 lbs per person. Wake up man! Your health problems and body fat are not an accident. Meanwhile, medical researchers are looking for the cause of diabetes so they can develop more sophisticated treatments.

Red grapes, red raisins, and red wine. Grapes are another one you must buy in August and early September when they are affordable to the average working person, i.e., $0.99 a pound instead of the usual $2.99 a pound. They are great for carb-loading on Fat Free Sunday, or HFFS (Half-day FFS), where you eat fruit "meals" for the first half of the day and the switch to 40 30 30 meals from about 3pm onward, for a milder carb-loading effect. For raisins, I always buy the Sunview brand jumbo organic black raisins. They are the best, juicy and plump, and some of them are huge. Sunview also sells red and green raisins. If you're not a raisin person, then try this brand, they're not like other raisins. Look for them at your healthfood store.

The NCD Chicken Alfredo™ recipe aliquots into 24 servings, and each serving comes with 1oz of red wine. You don't need 8-12 ounces, or an entire bottle, of red wine with dinner. Ask your liver if you don't believe me. Alcohol goes straight from the stomach to the liver for detoxification. Give it a rest. You can make the recipe in two batches of 12 and have 1-2 a day for the next week, or you can make three batches of 8 and have one meal a day, or you can do what I do and make all 24 at one time, and have Chicken Fettuccini Alfredo with Wine for breakfast, then four hours later for lunch, then a Flaxseed or Orange Shake at 15:00, and Chicken Fettuccini Alfredo with wine for dinner. It's an all day party. You might be thinking, "Don't you get bored of eating the same thing day after day?" No I don't. I enjoy the first meal as much as I enjoy the last one. The trick is, to build a

NCD ANNUAL MEAL PLAN ™

I've kept track of how often I like to eat a certain meal. The NCD Chicken Bowl™ is once per quarter, 4x a year, every 13 weeks. The NCD Steak Baked Beans™ and the NCD Teriyaki Chicken™ are each twice a year. And the NCD Chicken Alfredo™ is once a year. So by the time I finish the 24 meals, and 51 weeks has gone by, I'm ready for some Chicken Alfredo again. We'll look at building a NCD Annual Meal Plan™ in *12 Changes A Year*, but start thinking about it because once you've designed one, it takes the effort out of planning. You just look at your Annual Meal Plan chart and say, "Okay, next week I make this and this." Eventually, meal making and eating becomes sort of a mindless activity that you do just to allow yourself to focus 100% on living a productive happy life, so that you can be of service to your family and others.

At the end of my 24 Chicken Alfredo meals, I've had an entire 750mL bottle of red wine, 1oz at a time. I can walk into a supermarket and see red wine and feel nothing. I got it out of my system. Just like when I walk down the ice-cream aisle, I feel nothing. No pull. No draw. No urges. No cravings. I'm free. The Number Crunch Diet did it for me, and I believe it can do it for you too. As you eat the foods you desire, and don't eat the foods you don't desire, over time you will lose your desire for that food, and all foods, and simply eat to make your body perform, according to the needs of your Inner Divine Intelligence.

Chapter Endnotes
The fitness industry has their own spellings for certain words. This is done to facilitate and streamline their communications. Carb-load and carb-loading seem to be permanently hyphenated words on the internet.

high-glycemic shake – page 193
high glycemic corn – page 238
No I am not being inconsistent.
The first one is a, high-sugar shake, one&two three.
The second one is, High Sugar corn, One Two three.
The second one is an example of how the adjective "high" is trying to get some emphasis to describe "glycemic". So, hyphens speed you through a phrase, and no hyphens slow down the phrase. The same applies to comma use. At one time I was guilty of reading "the way I would read it", after reading a certain book, I was a bit frustrated when I got to the end, as I missed a lot of the meaning of many of the sentences. When I went back and read it "the way it was written", it was excellent.

This book's subtitle is really, "a step by step solution to alkaline deficiency", without hyphens. When you read the chapters step by step, you'll find the solution. Unfortunately, many people see the unhyphenated way as "incorrect" grammar. They look at things one way. JPM encourages you to be a broad thinker, and to see things as they are, without overlaying any preconceived templates. Sometimes, we think we know what the other person is trying to say, but we don't, and then we miss it.

CHAPTER 52

Phytonutrients Part 3

5. GREEN
Fruit
honeydew melon – summer
honeydew melon juice – see below
kiwifruit – fall
limes
lime juice
grapes & raisins
Vegetables
green beans
snap peas
snow peas
green peas – frozen
pea soup – canned or dried peas
asparagus – spring
artichoke – spring
bell pepper
celery
zucchini skin

Green beans are so easy to prepare. Wash them, cut off the ends, boil until ¾ done, then aliquot each pound of beans into four 4oz servings, I use the pyrex small rectangle with the red lid. Let the beans cool and the moisture evaporate before putting the lid on and refrigerating. Then, as a snack or as part of a meal, pull out your green beans and snack on them before you begin eating your meal, and then have a few with your meal, and there you have it. You just ate four ounces of green vegetable with your lunch.

The NCD Orange Chicken™ uses boxed orange chicken from S&F, but it's a good brand with no preservatives or colors, and the protein content is pretty good. I add extra chopped chicken breast and some white rice, topped with 14g of hemp seeds, and the mandarin orange sauce. It's delicious and satisfies my desire for orange chicken. However, there isn't enough sauce for the green beans. I tried adding the green beans to the recipe and it diluted out the sauce, thus, diluting out the flavor, and the fun. So now I have boiled green beans on the side. Boiled green beans are delicious, if, you don't overcook them. Remove them at ¾ doneness and let them finish cooking off heat. I have recorded the exact number of minutes so that my beans come out al dente, soft but firm. Then just eat them like french fries. They are practically the same shape and texture. Seriously. It almost feels like you're eating french fries. Make a plate of al-dente green beans and a plate of french fries and see which one your family eats. I will bet they'll reach for the green beans, because that's what the body wants. There's nothing nutritious about french fries. We just eat them because we see them everywhere, it's ingrained in our cultural psyche, hence, we go through life semi-aware, eating and doing things on autopilot much of the time.

Snap Peas. This is such an easy way to get a raw green vegetable. Buy three bags of snap peas, they used to come in 16oz bags, but they are making the packages smaller and raising the prices so that we don't notice that the price of food has doubled in recent years. The metric system for buying food is a pricing gimmick. 454 grams of turkey sounds like a lot of turkey, so let's charge a lot of money for it, but it's just one pound, which doesn't sound like much. Next they'll be selling us gasoline for our cars by the liter! I place all three bags of snap peas in a big bowl and wash and strain them three times. Transfer them to a towel, fold it over and by holding the ends of the towel, swing it back-and-forth to towel dry the snap peas. Now, aliquot them into nine medium pyrex bowls with the red lids, 4oz per bowl. You just made yourself nine 4oz servings of snap peas. Place them by your computer and snack on them while you're working to be sure you get your daily Green.

Frozen peas and pea soup, the NCD has recipes for these, and pea soup is a great way of obtain protein from plants instead of from animals all the time. Technically, dried peas are beans, but then you have peas that are vegetables, and peas that are beans, so I put the bean-peas together with the vegetable-peas, since they are both green in color.

Asparagus. See the NCD Buffalo Chicken™.

Artichoke is included as part of the NCD Tuna Pasta Salad™. I originally placed artichokes under Yellow for their heart color, but visually they just didn't fit. You can eat some of the flesh from the leaves as it does contain antioxidants, and Green color.   The farmers that grew my artichokes have been growing artichokes from the same plants stocks passed down from generation-to-generation for nearly 100 years. Do you see how this is different than buying herbicide-resistant genetically-modified seeds?

Bell Pepper.   Here is another great way to get a green raw vegetable. Buy six beautiful fresh green bell peppers. If they are wrinkled a bit, you won't enjoy them. Your Internal Intelligence can tell that they are beginning to spoil. Wash and dry them three times to remove pesticides. That means, wash in hot water, then towel dry, and repeat, wash in hot water, and towel dry, last time, wash in hot water, and towel dry. You won't enjoy them if there is pesticide residue on the surface, and your Divine Intelligence won't like it either. The towel drying after each wash will ensure that you have removed those nasty glued-on pesticide sprays.   Toss the towel in the laundry basket. Now, cut out the stem and slice the pepper in half and scoop out the insides. Holding the pepper in one hand or by placing it on a cutting board, slice it into strips. Add 4oz of bell pepper strips to a small pyrex rectangle, cover with the red lid and repeat until you have sliced up all six bell peppers. You should now have about ten servings of 4oz green bell pepper.

Snack on this before a meal or as part of a meal if the recipe doesn't include a vegetable.

Several of the NCD recipes don't have a vegetable as part of the meal, and so the green beans on the side, or the snap peas, or the sliced bell pepper, or 4oz cherry tomatoes, will be your vegetable.

Buy 3, 12oz packs of organic cherry tomatoes, wash and drain 3x, then towel swing dry. Organic only requires one towel drying since no pesticides are used. Aliquot the cherry tomatoes into 8oz SKS glass jars with screw caps or extra-small pyrex bowls, 4oz per serving. That's your red vegetable for the day, and for the next 8 days, 3pk x 12oz = 36oz divided by 4oz = 9 servings. Also for Red, you could do the 6 bell peppers using 3 red and 3 green.

Celery. Cut off the ends and wash and drain the stalks 3x with hot water. Cut in three-inch lengths and fill your SKS 8oz jars with the sticks. Cap and refrigerate. Do half celery and half carrot sticks if you want. Don't add water like they do in the supermarkets as the water takes away the flavor and nutrients from the vegetable. Recall that water is an absorber, a dissolver. So then you drain off the water to eat your celery and carrots and the celery sodium and carrot minerals go down the drain. Instead, use the SKS jar with screw cap and the celery and carrots will stay fresh, sealed in the airtight container without the need for water.

Cucumber and Organic Green Zucchini. Cut off the ends, wash and towel dry 3x to remove pesticides, or 1x if organic. Cut them in 3-inch lengths, and then turn each 3-inch section on its end and cut top-to-bottom, left-to-right, (+), into quarters, sticks. Your SKS 8oz glass jar is 3 and 1/8th inches deep, so your cucumber sticks will fix perfectly to the top. You can also do the following. Cut off the ends, then put the cucumber into the 8oz SKS jar and cut it by running the knife along the rim of the jar. Remove it and cut it in quarters. Repeat repeat repeat. This cutting technique allows you to have cucumber sticks that are the exact height of the jar, and therefore, less air and longer expiration times. English cucumbers are about 13-14 inches long, so when you cut off the ends you have

12 inches remaining, and this cuts into 3 3 3 3 inches. You will enjoy your vegetable sticks more when they look professionally prepared. Plus, people will admire what you're eating. Picture an 8oz glass jar with a smooth white cap filled with green-and-white cucumber or zucchini sticks all the same height, at the level of the rim. This is quite different than a bag of chips. People will take notice. When they do, refer them to where they can purchase this book so I can reach out to more people.

Each 8oz SKS jar will hold four cucumber or 4-5 zucchini sticks, and this is a 4oz serving. So there you have another great way to get a raw vegetable, free calories, and a pat on the back. The sks-bottle.com 8oz glass jars seem like there were custom designed for vegetable sticks, they're the perfect size.

If you want a hot vegetable, cut the ends off the zucchini, then quarter it; run your knife through the center, parallel to the cutting board, and then through the center again, but perpendicular to the cutting board, then slice it from end to end in one-inch increments. Aliquot your zucchini chunks into small pyrex bowls, 4oz each, cover with the lids and refrigerate. Two pounds of zucchini should yield about eight servings, as the ends that you cut off and discard are thin. The math is, 2x16oz=32oz ÷4oz=8 servings. To cook them, just place the bowl with the 4oz of zucchini in the microwave, no need to add any water, and microwave for 60 seconds. They come out perfect. Al dente, firm but soft. I eat them plain, but you can sprinkle a little parmesan cheese on top, or better yet, a dash sprinkle from your curry or turmeric shaker.

Kiwifruit, eat them alone on FFS or as the fruit portion of a meal. Just be sure to buy them fresh. The skins should be tight all over with no wrinkles, especially around the stem, in fact, the skin should give the impression that it's going to burst open because it's so tight and taut. When you find them like this, they will feel heavy for their size, nice. Good kiwifruit is hard to find as the majority of the time they lack that kiwi flavor. If you get home and find you've got a winner! go back to the store as soon as possible before they're all sold out and buy a bunch more. Then peel them, slice them up into a bowl and enjoy that zingy kiwi flavor! A one-pound container or bag of kiwifruit, six medium kiwifruit, is about 250 calories, perfect as part of your FFS or HFFS.

Flavor makes such a difference. Not only is the nutrient content at its maximum when the flavor is at its maximum, but the look on people's faces when they eat it will bring joy to your heart. We've all seen vine-ripened tomatoes at the store, beautiful-looking, delicious-tasting tomatoes cut from the vine instead of picked from the stem. Well, one time, and one time only, Albertson's had vine-ripened peaches with the stems still attached. Wow, were they good. People at work had one and then they'd come back and have another and then they'd come back again saying, "Those are so good, I just have to have another." What's happening is, their Divine Intelligence has recognized nutrition. Nutrition that it gave up looking for ten years ago. So now it says, "Yes! Peach nutrients! Keep 'em coming!" If only we could have all of our produce cut from the vine instead of picked from the stem.

Honeydew Melon. Buy this in the summer when it's in season and on sale and eat one or two to get your body stores stocked up on honeydew nutrients until next season. For honeydew-melon juice, follow the same steps as for the cantaloupe but use 1/3 of the rind with the seeds and flesh.

NCD Melon Juices™ with the seeds and flesh, plus:
Cantaloupe   use all the rind
Honeydew   use 1/3 of the rind
Watermelon   use 1/4 of the rind

I encourage you to make these juices every season at least one time for each melon per year. They are loaded with good plant-color nutrition and a whole host of other properties that your DI will thank you for. Aside from these, you should be consuming Green on a weekly rotational basis, just pick one from the list, make 7-10 servings for the week, and then switch to a different one the following week. Leafy Greens are a special Green and so they have their own separate category.

CHAPTER 53

Phytonutrients Part 4

LEAFY GREENS
cilantro
kale
spinach
spring mix
swiss chard
wheatgrass shot

Cilantro. This is one of my favorite greens and you might ask why it is that I call it a leafy green. For its detox properties. I don't want to make claims about cilantro, but one author wrote that after being in the Gulf War in 1990-2, the smoke and toxic air made him so sick he thought he was not going to recover. After trying a list of remedies, he stated that it was eating lots of fresh cilantro that cleaned out his lungs and restored his health.

Buy one big bunch or two small bunches, preferably organic, but most importantly FRESH. Freshness of your leafy greens is your top priority. Never buy them if they are not fresh. Try another store, or go with spinach or kale, or have the wheatgrass shot. Triple-wash the cilantro in hot water. Fill a large bowl with hot water, then "dip-wash" six times, discard the water and repeat two more times. Flick off the excess water, pull off the leaves from the stems, leaving a little of the stems is fine, and place the leaves in a bowl with lid and refrigerate. The faster you can wash them and get them into the refrigerator, the longer they will last without spoiling. If you do it fast enough, they should stay fresh 6-7 days. Have one handful each morning first thing when you wake up. If you choose to wash in the sink, be sure that the sink is clean and well-rinsed to remove soaps and detergents. Wiping the surfaces of the sink with a towel is an effective way to remove soap residues.

If you get up at 06:00, be sure to have your greens by 06:10, or 06:15 at the latest. This way, if the rest of your day sucks, then at least you got your greens in, so it wasn't a complete disaster. Also in the morning, before breakfast, is a good time to have a shot of Noni juice or Acai or Goji puree. Now you've done two good things for your health and you haven't even had breakfast.

Kale and Swiss Chard. Buy one bunch on the weekend and prep it for Monday and the week. Bagged chopped kale tastes stronger and not very good in my opinion, so always buy fresh looking (and if possible, organic) bunched kale and swiss chard. Wash it 3x in hot water, dipping 6x, drain and repeat two more times. Flick off the excess water and place the leaves in a large bowl with lid and refrigerate. Kale and Swiss Chard leaves can tolerate hot-water washings much more than cilantro. Have one big leaf or two small leaves per day and finish it by Sunday so you can begin Monday with a new leafy green. Again, have it when you first wake up so as to get your leafy green out of the way. Chew it thoroughly and it won't come back on you.

Spinach. Kale and Spinach are high in Lutein for your vision, this is why they began selling carrot juice with greens, for additional vision support. Buy two 6oz bags or one 12oz bag or one bunch of spinach if it looks fresh. The bagged spinach is usually fresh and tastes fresh. Add them to a big bowl of hot water, wash and drain them 3x using a colander. Be quick so they don't wilt. If the bag says it's triple-washed, then one wash is sufficient. You will know when you go to eat it if it still has pesticides on it, gurgle gurgle. Then you'll stop eating spinach because you had a bad experience. If you see dirt or suds during the first wash, then wash and drain 3x. A salad spinner works great for removing excess water, spin in two batches and then add them to a large bowl with lid and refrigerate. Place one big handful in a cereal bowl and munch on them as you are getting ready for work and making breakfast.

If by Thursday the leaves are looking a bit wilted, then double your portion and finish them by the next day. You had them in the hot water too long, or your refrigerator isn't staying cold, or it's not set cold enough. I keep two thermometers inside my refrigerator, one on the top so I can see it when I open the door, and one on the bottom shelf door. Adjust the thermostat so that the temperature stays close to 0°C 32°F. Don't worry, your food won't freeze. This is an additional way to extend the expiration of your meals and food.

Keep your refrigerator's temperature at 0°C for extended food-expiration.™

Spring Mix, the easiest of all to prepare, as there is none! Go to Walmart and buy the Organic Spring Mix 10oz 284g. Just eat a handful each morning straight from the container. It says "triple washed and ready to enjoy" on the label, and I've never had a bad experience from not washing it. It's $4.98÷7=$0.71 per serving, so twice the cost of what you'll pay for kale or spinach, but perfect if you don't have time to prep food. If you open it on Monday, it won't last until Sunday, so plan to finish it in 4-5 days, as you don't want to be eating wilted greens or be throwing away your money.

Wheat Grass Shots are available at Lassen's my local healthfood store. They take organic wheatgrass and squish it through a vegetable grinder and out comes a bright green liquid that they collect in a small plastic "shot glass" type of cup. Next time I might bring my own GLASS shot glass to get away from the taste of plastic. I've come to enjoy the clean taste of drinking from glass so much that I've become a Plastiphobe™. The NCD encourages you to become a Plastiphobe too. Try using the following words in a sentence the next time you're talking to someone.

Plastiphobe   Plastiphobia   Plastiphobic   Plastiphobism

NCD Plastiphobism™ – the practice of avoiding plastic containers! A person who believes in using nontoxic environmentally-friendly glass containers whenever possible. One who also avoids waxy-paper cups, styrofoam cups, and use-once throw-away containers.

Anyway, for $1.49 per ounce you can get a good dose of green plant juice and chlorophyll from the WGS. Chlorophyll is what gives plants their green color, soaking up energy from the sun and converting it into energy for the plant. You can add this energy to your body by consuming foods with chlorophyll, and the best way to achieve this is through leafy greens. So, if I haven't had my leafy greens this week, I do the 1oz wheatgrass shot, which I consider equal to a week's worth of leafy greens. Follow it with a shot of water to wash it down as there's no sugar in it and it tastes pretty much like what you would expect your lawn to taste like.

NCD Leafy Greens™ protocol
week 1 Cilantro
week 2 Kale or Swiss Chard
week 3 Spinach
week 4 Spring Mix
Wheat Grass Shot, one per week, if you didn't have time to make your leafy greens or you didn't buy them because they didn't look fresh.

CHAPTER 54

Phytonutrients Part 5

So the color foods we have so far are, white, yellow, orange, red, green, leafy green, and the last one is purple blue black, PBB.

PURPLE BLUE BLACK
Solids
Fruit
bing cherries – August
blackberries – summer, year round, and frozen
black current juice – store bought
acai puree juice – bioinnovations.net
Vegetable
beets – fresh, canned okay
Exterior
Fruit
blueberries – summer, and frozen
prune plums – summer, and dried
grapes, raisins, and juice – August, and year round
plums – summer
Vegetables
cabbage
onion
eggplant

Bing cherries are a great source of black, just be sure to buy them during that two-week window in August as they will be firm and fresh. If you get there late and they are a little soft, DON'T BUY THEM! The flesh and skin are so deep dark purple-black that you can't see the spoiled areas. You will only find out later that they were starting to spoil, and you won't like how you feel. So pay attention to the weekly flyers that come in the mail, or just be sure to visit your local supermarket once a week during the summer months and look for them. There's nothing better than fresh firm in-season produce, and there's nothing worse than produce that's beginning to spoil.

Blackberries are available year round and the price it about the same all year. I often buy four 18oz containers, divide them into five servings of 410g 14.5oz, and with the fiber subtracted you have a 250-calorie solid black. Have them on FFS, HFFS, the NCD One Fruit 'Meal', or as the carb/dessert portion of a meal.

Beets. This is a special vegetable. First of all, it's the only vegetable in the PBB category that's purple all the way through. Red cabbage, that looks purple, is white on the inside, and it's hard to eat significant amounts because it has a stronger taste than green cabbage. Same for Bermuda purple "red" onion, it's white on the inside and you can't eat a significant amount. Eggplant rind is black, but the interior is white, and so not a good source for purple blue black.

This is an interesting discovery. That is, there seems to be one primary vegetable in each color group. By "primary" I mean common, and one that you could eat every day, and has a solid color all the way through. The green color group has two common solids.

WHITE	cucumber, 4oz are free
	potatoes are white but they contain starch calories
YELLOW	bell pepper, 4oz are free
	corn is yellow, but it has starch calories
ORANGE	carrots, 4oz are free
	pumpkin has solid orange color, but not as popular
	sweet potatoes, starch vegetable therefore not free

RED	tomatoes, 4oz are free
	red bell peppers aren't as popular
GREEN	green beans, 4oz are free
GREEN	snap peas, 4oz are free
	green peas are a starch vegetable
	asparagus and artichoke are seasonal, less popular
	celery, part of carrots and celery sticks
PBB	beets, 4oz are free

Beets and carrots have about 35-37 net calories in a 4oz serving but their benefits are so tremendous that they are considered free. Beets are blood cleansers, blood detoxifiers. Any time you have a serving of beets you get a pat on BOTH sides of your back. Clean Blood = Clean Body. Dirty blood, dirty body. Ask someone when the last time it was that they ate beets. For many people, beets is not even on their radar screen and has never crossed their minds. You don't see them in restaurants, except in a single crock in the salad bar. Bring beets to the front of your awareness and start eating them. The NCD Beets™ recipe will get you started eating canned beets right away, and then you can switch to fresh beets, a bit more work but well worth it. Consider beets the same as tomatoes carrots and green beans, common.

So our seven solid-color vegetables, all 4oz servings, all free, are:
NCD Color Vegetable™ protocol
1. Cucumber (or organic non-GMO zucchini)
2. Bell Pepper (yellow, or 50/50 yellow & green)
3. Carrots (including carrot & celery sticks)
4. Tomatoes
5. Green Beans
6. Snap Peas
7. Beets
For celery, I sometimes just pick up a stalk at the supermarket if it looks firm and fresh, take it home, wash it, and snack on it over the remainder of the day. So, celery is another one that you can prepare and have for free.

And our free 3oz citrus "vegetable" is Ruby Red Grapefruit.

We also have our four estrogen-lowering testosterone-boosting vegetables, one serving per day on a four-week rotation cycle.

NCD Four T Vegetable™ protocol
week 1 broccoli
week 2 brussel sprouts
week 3 cauliflower
week 4 coleslaw

Along with our
NCD Leafy Greens™ protocol
week 1 cilantro
week 2 kale or swiss chard
week 3 spinach
week 4 spring mix
        or WGS

So your day might look like this.
06:00 up
06:10 leafy greens – free
07:00 Breakfast 500cal
09:00 cucumber 4oz – free
10:00 Snack 250cal
12:00 Lunch 500cal
15:00 broccoli with 5g sprinkle of parmesan – free
16:00 Flaxseed Shake 500cal
18:00 Dinner 500cal
21:00 cherry tomatoes 4oz – free
22:00 lights out

For additional color and nutrition, include a shot of Noni, Acai, Goji, or Mangosteen after your leafy greens. Noni fruit is grown on the mineral-rich volcanic soil on the island of Hawaii, not on the mineral-depleted soils of, well, I won't say where.

Total calories is 2250, 4 meals x 500 plus 1 snack x 250. We had our daily handful of leafy greens, we had a White, we had a T-veg, and we had a Red. We ate all day, and came in at 250 calories under for the day. Remarkable!

If you did 45 minutes of the NCD Recalibration Exercise™ at a moderate pace or 30 minutes at a fast pace, that's another 250 calories. So the total under for the day is 500 calories, or one pound of butter fat off your body each week. You could easily keep this up for six months to a year and drop 25-50 pounds. No rice cakes, no tofu, and no plain salads with breadsticks.

If you wanted to lose weight a little faster at the beginning because maybe you are really motivated, just sporadically skip some of the carbs in a meal. For example, if you are having the NCD Roast Beef Sandwich™ that we talked about earlier, just omit the raisins from the three squares of dark-chocolate almond bar. For the NCD Turkey Cheese & Crackers™, omit the pear for dessert, or just have half of it. Just omit a small portion of the carbs of any meal, but do it SPORADICALLY so that your body doesn't notice that you're cutting additional carbs. If you get too carried away and start omitting some of the carbs at every meal, then your body will catch on to the trick and say, "Hey! You've been cutting my carbs!" Then it goes on a carb-eating binge to catch up and get itself back to its old homeostatic weight again.

If you're a male and you require 2750 calories a day, then make your 10:00 snack a 500 calorie meal in the above example. Your total calories will be 2500, 250 under. Then do 30 minutes of "cross-country-ski" walking on a treadmill at 4.0 mph each day and that will burn another 250+ calories, so you are losing 500 per day, one pound of body fat per week. You won't even notice it. You could continue like this for months until you reach your desired weight. Then, to prevent yourself from becoming too thin, yes, I said too thin, add a 250cal snack at 20:00, two hours before bed. Remember, a snack is 40% carbs 30% fat 30% protein, not a bag of chips. Meals and Snacks are all 40 30 30.

Each person's needs will be different, some will want weight loss, some will want weight gain, some just want a good healthy plan for weight maintenance. The way to do that is to count calories by counting Pre-Counted Meals™, and the Number Crunch Diet allows you to do this easily without a calculator. Six meals a day, 3000 calories, 5 meals, 2500, 4 meals 2000, 5 meals and a snack, 2750, 4 meals and 2 snacks, 2500. You've got it!

Plus it encourages you to eat the Free vegetables, starting your day with one of the four leafy greens, kale, spinach, spring mix, cilantro, then have a primary color, 4oz of cucumber, carrot, yellow & green bell peppers, a sliced vine-ripened tomato, or 4oz of cherry tomatoes, 4oz of green beans, or 4oz of snap peas, 4oz of beets, a T vegetable with a little sprinkle of parmesan cheese, and 3oz of grapefruit. You eat every two to three hours, and avoid going more than four hours without eating. Recalibrate your hormones, metabolism, and brain function, with cross-country-ski walking. Eat what you want, checking with your Divine Intelligence when making decisions, no more external eating. You break free from any food addictions by stopping the consumption of food chemicals, as well as avoiding food poisons. And having done all that, you'll be well-on-your-way to being in control of your body weight, appetite, and health, for the rest of your life.

The Number Crunch Diet
a New and Unique approach to weight management

CHAPTER 55

CLO

Cod Liver Oil. At one time I worked as a bartender and waiter, and one of the things customers would do at the bar was to have a shot of alcohol in front of them, put their arms behind their back, then they would bend over, grab the shot glass with their mouth, and throw their head back. The crowd would roar and the person's face would turn red. I never did this, I just made easy money off those that did.

Fast-forward 20 years, and this same technique came to me in a flash as a way to get a hefty dose of cod liver oil without letting the oil sit in your mouth and activating your taste buds. Hence, the NCD CLO Shot™. The 1oz SKS small glass jars work perfectly for this. But first, a history on CLO.

In 2008 I purchased 12 bottles of cod liver oil, 8oz per bottle, so 3 quarts CLO total, from Iceland Health, www.icelandhealth.com. I had been taking CLO in small amounts sporadically, a teaspoon or two here-and-there for about two years prior and not seen any benefit. Then I went BIG. One ounce, the NCD CLO Shot™. This is when I saw immediate results.

I consumed eight 8oz bottles that year, that's half a gallon of cod liver oil. This is serious CLO therapy. But here's what I documented. "Soft Thick Hair" "Mobile Lubricated Joints" "Tons of Energy" "20-Years Younger" "No Muscle Soreness or Pain".

This was an amazing discovery for me. Some days I felt so good, I would take two shots a day, that's a quarter-of-a-cup of cod liver oil. The most I ever took in one day was four 1oz shots, half a cup of cod liver oil. That was the day I noted that my joints were mobile and lubricated with no pain and I felt 20-years younger. I then bought another 12 bottles, 3 quarts from icelandhealth.com.

Later, in 2010 I went to place my order for a third time and the product was off their website. I emailed customer service. No reply. I called them, and they just said they don't sell it anymore. Now, all they sell is fish oil in capsules.

Hm. That's interesting.

One typical softgel of CLO is equal to about a ½t of the liquid. The typical cost for 30 softgels is about $25, which is equal to about 15t or 5T (tablespoons) or 2.5 volume ounces of the liquid.

The 8oz bottle of CLO that I used to buy was $7.99. If you purchased 12 bottles, the price was 20% off, so $6.39 per bottle.

In order to obtain 8oz of CLO from the softgels, you would have to purchase about 3.2 containers of the 30-count softgels. The math is, 3.2x30=96 half teaspoons, divided by 2 = 48 teaspoons, divided by 3 = 16 Tablespoons, divided by 2 = 8 ounces.

1oz = 2T = 6t   1T = 3t

The cost would be, 3.2 x $25 = $80.

So, I used to pay $7.99 or $6.39 for eight ounces of liquid cod liver oil, and now to get that same eight ounces, I would have to buy 3.2 containers of the softgels for $80.

This is ten times as much money. Pure Greed.

So now I buy the 12oz bottle of Twinlab brand CLO from www.swansonvitamins.com for $8.97 and free shipping.

Thank you Swanson's Vitamins and Twinlab.

If you are buying CLO in capsule form, you are being ripped off.™

The first way is, the small amount in the capsule is not enough to have any real effect. You would have to take 6 softgels just to get one tablespoon of liquid CLO, which is how much they took in the old days. If you took 6 softgels a day, you would finish that $25 container in 5 days. If you took 6 softgels a day, equal to about one tablespoon of CLO, for one month, you would have spent $150, times 12 months equals $1800 a year for cod liver oil capsules.

Fish oil is now the number-one selling supplement on the market. I wonder why? Huge profit margins maybe.

So, number one, the softgels are equal to about a 1/2t of liquid oil. Too little to be effective, in my opinion. And number two, the price is roughly ten-times more for the softgels than for the liquid cod liver oil.

Additionally, they are making them in all sorts of varieties with added ingredients like resveratrol and CoQ10 and giving them names like, fish oil for your joints, fish oil for your heart, one for your vision, one for your immune system. This is deception at its worst, in my opinion. Shame shame. You take CLO for the DHA and EPA, that's the reason why you take it. So don't waste your money on designer-CLO products, and never buy the capsules, only the liquid.

Now, please don't take bits-and-pieces of what I say and switch to liquid CLO and a month later it tastes fishy. You have to read this entire chapter and store the liquid CLO airtight in sealed 1oz jars, because what do we know about CLO? What? I can't hear you, what? It spoils quickly due to the unstable "U" shape of the fatty acids DHA and EPA. So, if you don't plan on storing the liquid properly, then yes, you should buy the capsules.

In my opinion, I believe that they are marketing cod liver oil in capsules now instead of liquid so that doctors can prescribe them, "Take two capsules in the morning, take two capsules in the evening." You don't need a doctor to tell you how much cod liver oil to take, just picture your grandparents and how they took it. Your grandparents poured plain CLO from an amber bottle onto a spoon. The CLO provided them with the essential DHA and EPA that they needed, and that we still need today. It did not contain resveratrol, CoQ10, or other fancy-sounding formulations. The next generations stopped this good habit and now we're all deficient. I certainly was as I consumed half a gallon in one year.

The NCD CLO Shot™ is a good dose of CLO, it's exactly 1.2 fluid ounces or 2.4 tablespoons. This is equal to about 14.4 softgels.

A very-popular heart doctor said that he takes up to 16 softgels per day. Someone needs to introduce him to the NCD CLO Shot™. I can't imagine how your digestive system would deal with all of those gelatin capsules.

The 30-softgels-for-$25 example is almost $1 per softgel, $0.83 each. So if the cardiologist is taking up to 16 per day, he's spending $13.33 per day or $400 a month on fish oil. Luckily he can afford it, but I doubt this is the case for most people.

When a doctor gets on television and advises the viewers to take 8 to 10 to 12 or even 16 capsules of fish oil a day, this is deception at its worst and shameful, especially when sold alongside of Christianity. Yes, you need big doses of CLO, but not from capsules. Jesus got angry only one time in the Bible, when the money changers were thieving off the people.

The consumer is being cheated by overpriced small-volume softgel fish oil capsules. When what you need is a sufficient volume of fish oil to get the effects of taking fish oil. This is available in affordable liquid bottles. Additionally, the benefit is the fish oil itself, not the fancy additions.™ You heard it here first.

There are some tricks to taking fish oil so that you don't have digestive issues. The shot goes down good if you do it correctly. The NCD does have salmon recipes but I don't consume them often enough and this is why I do the CLO Shots, to make up for my low fish oil diet. And if you've never taken CLO and you've not eaten much salmon over the past 10-20 years, you are likely low on DHA and EPA and so you may need several CLO Shots per week for a year or more to get you stocked up. Then one shot a week for maintenance, I take mine on Saturdays.

From 2006 to 2009 I consumed more than a gallon of cod liver oil. That's deficiency. You would need to take approximately 1536 softgels or about 51 containers of 30-count softgels to equal one gallon of CLO. Those 51 containers would cost $1275. I paid ~$102 for the same volume by purchasing the liquid.

The Twinlab-CLO label has one ingredient, cod liver oil. Nice. That's all I want.   That's what has the EPA and DHA, Eicosapentaenoic Acid and Docosahexaenoic Acid, these are fatty acid chains with 5 and 6 double bonds respectively. Your omega-3 flaxseed fatty acid has 3 double bonds, and your omega-9 olive oil avocado and peanuts has one double bond. Animal fat and coconut oil have no double bonds, they are straight-line fatty acid chains, rigid, stiff, inflexible. And as a reminder, we don't eat the other oils, burnt, trans, and refined omega-6.

The significance of DHA and EPA is that they convert to PG3, series three prostaglandins, "Fast-Acting Hormones". These PG3 hormones are responsible for all those good things we hear about, like calming inflammation, lowering blood pressure, and improving circulation. Could it be that all of these inflammation-related diseases, high blood pressure, and circulatory problems, are simply due to a decades-long lack of dietary fish oil?

Hmm. Ponder that for a moment. Maybe reread it.

PG3 is not to be confused with PG1, that has similar anti-inflammatory effects but is synthesized from the GLA found highest in Borage Oil (see Chapter 49).

For a double dose of anti-inflammatory, take both CLO & GLA.™

The NCD Triple Anti-Inflammatory™
1. take CLO
2. take Borage Oil
3. stop taking refined omega-6 oil, man-made oil, and fryer oil

As mentioned before, a small percentage of our omega-3 flaxseed will convert to fish oil DHA and EPA, so this is a nice backup, and omega-3 flax, chia, hemp, and walnuts, is the only fat that can do this.

And just a quick review, the other two dietary fats, omega-9 OAP and saturated animal and coconut oil, are good and fine, but not essential. The two that we need to seek out and consume in our daily and weekly diets are, Omega-3 Flax and Cod Liver Oil.

The Twinlab label says "Quality Tested For Purity" and "Molecularly Distilled" and the bottle is free of air, (nitrogen flushed), to prevent oxidation and rancidity. There is a warning to pregnant mothers and people on medication to consult with their healthcare provider, which has been stated several times in this book, that people seeing a doctor are under the care of their doctor and not following a selfcare book. As most of us know, fish oil can "thin" your blood, making blood clotting slower, so, if you are on coumadin or plavix or oral heparin or aspirin, anticoagulants and antiplatelet aggregators, you could potentially bleed out. Your doctor knows this, that's why you consult with your doctor if you are on medications. People with bad diets and who are overweight are likely walking around with slightly "sludgy" blood, so a little "thinning" is probably a good thing for them, but this is a broad generalization. Read the label and proceed accordingly.

Ah. I just returned from having my weekly NCD CLO Shot™. The 1.2 fluid ounces of CLO that I have once a week averages out to about 1t per day or about 2 softgels per day. This is my maintenance amount, you will need much much more if you've never taken it before and you haven't been eating fatty fish.

The NCD CLO Shot Aliquoting Procedure™
Divide the 12oz bottle of Twinlab CLO into ten 1oz SKS glass jars, filling them to the brim. You will want to bend down so you can see the jar rims at eye level. Fill them to the brim, full to the top, flat. Now, carefully place the cap on top and screw it on hand-tight. This way, there is no air inside and they will last for the full ten weeks without going rancid. Store them in the refrigerator.

On your CLO-Shot day, remove it from the refrigerator in the morning when you get up so that it warms to room temperature. This is the key. Never take CLO straight from the refrigerator as it will not go down well. People store their fish-oil capsules in the refrigerator, this is good, but then they open the container and pop one or two capsules at 0-4°C and wonder why it comes back on them. To avoid fish burps, follow the NCD CLO Rule #1.™

STORE IT COLD, TAKE IT AT ROOM TEMPERATURE™

Also, don't take it near mealtimes. Use the NCD CLO Rule #2.™

CLO 2 HOURS AFTER AND 2 HOURS BEFORE MEALS™

So, if I get up at 07:00, I take my CLO Shot out of the refrigerator to warm up. Then, breakfast at 08:00, the CLO Shot at 10:00, and lunch at 12 noon. This way there is no interference, and it goes down without you even noticing it. Just pick the "shot" glass up with your mouth and swing your head back and take one big swallow. Follow it with a couple of saliva swallows, and that's it. In 15 minutes you won't even remember having taken it.

The cost per shot is $0.90. If I was to buy the equivalent amount in softgel form the cost would be about $12. This is great DHA and EPA supplementation and makes up for my lack of being able to pull fresh wild salmon out of my backyard river. Just be sure to aliquot it as above, store it in the refrigerator, take it at room temperature, 2 hours away from meals, and use it within 10 weeks.

I consume 12 ounces per quarter, so if I am consistent and take 10 shots in 10 weeks, then I get 3 weeks off, and then begin again. In the summertime I slack a bit because of the warm weather, but by the end of the year I have had at least 32oz or one quart, and that's good cod liver oil insurance in my opinion.

Clearly, no one can accuse me of giving vague advice. Everything I suggest here, I do, having created a system for doing it for myself, the reader can follow it and do the same. There are other things that I hope to cover in future publications, things like, making your own turkey and beef jerky, sprouting fresh living alfalfa sprouts, and making your own vanilla extract from vanilla beans and vodka. So I hope you'll join me when you're ready for your Master's Degree in Number Crunchology – *12 Changes A Year*.

So take your 1oz SKS glass jars and your 12oz Twinlab CLO to your next family gathering and do NCD CLO Shots™ at the table two hours before dinner. And don't be surprised if after a while your hair gets thicker and your joints feel younger.

EPA = Eicosapentaenoic = i-co-sa-penta-en-no-ic Acid
DHA = Docosahexaenoic = doe-co-sa-hexa-en-no-ic Acid

Use those words in a sentence at your next employee potluck and you'll gain a whole new look of respect.

And then when they ask you why you don't refer to them as Omega-3s. Tell them, flax, chia, and hemp seeds have three double bonds whereas EPA and DHA have 5 and 6 double bonds. They're not the same molecules, and although they have overlapping roles, they also have uniquely different functions.

Chapter Endnote
Say "soap". Now drop the "s", oh-p, or OAP. This may help you to remember the three omega-9s, or, the oap fats.

Addendum

I don't normally shop for margarine, so I hadn't noticed this. The makers of margarine, Imperial etc., have changed the name of their product to Vegetable Oil Spread. How bad is it that you have to change the name of your product because of government warnings telling us that trans fat is health damaging fat.

So, "Vegetable Oil Spread" is fully hydrogenated, instead of the old partially and fully hydrogenated mixture. It can still contain trans fat, but say "zero" on the label, because 0.4 rounds down to 0. So if you buy a 5 lb tub of VOS, and it has 160 servings, that's 160 x 0.4 = 64 grams of trans fat or 576 calories of trans fat per container.

I use the words "margarine" and "trans fat" interchangeable. Well, just for the record, it's more accurately called now "vegetable oil spread" and "fully hydrogenated oil". Probably they use these long names so that authors will stop writing bad things about them because the name is three words long and too cumbersome.

They can run but they can't hide, they can change the name from margarine to vegetable oil spread, but it's still margarine to me. And fully hydrogenated is still hydrogenated. If you can find anywhere in the Bible or in the history books of the people eating "vegetable oil spread" then go ahead and eat it. That's my advice.

The NCD says No to Hydrogenated Plant Oils, regardless of the name that they give it, and regardless of whether it's fully or partially hydrogenated.

CHAPTER 56

the MIXED DIET

There's another common diet program that keeps being repeated by various authors, and it's the mixed approach. You do three days of Atkins, little or no carbs, followed by one day of eating chocolate cupcakes. Seriously. This is what's being touted on television by a doctor and his new diet book.

Don't kid yourself. If you think that you are not going to go overboard on your "cupcake day" you are living in dreamland. There is just no substitution for consistent good nutrition and calorie counting. You are just delaying results and wasting precious time and energy by following more bad advice thinking that "maybe this is the answer".

Here again, we have science students with more brains than the author of this doctor's diet book. Actually, that's not quite correct. The doctor knows how to make money off the public, just tell them something they want to hear. It's the consumers that buy his book, they are the ones being fooled. The diet doctor wants to sell books and make money from his viewers, and since it works, he's actually quite smart. Honest and noble, not really. But business smart, yes.

The NCD principles are based on eating carbs with every meal, eating fat with every meal, and then making sure that your protein is there and at 30%. If you skimp on the protein, then your meal starts to resemble a dessert, fats and carbs. That's a recipe for weight gain.

By staying on a 40% carb 30% fat 30% protein meal formula, you have a complete meal, and you won't need to "jumpstart your metabolism" out of a plateau because your energy will be in the medium-steady range, or better, your entire day every day.

Isn't that the ideal way to be? Stable Energy. Stable Mood.

If you do at some point hit a plateau, here's what you do. And this happened to me. My body fat had gotten low, and I wanted it to go lower still, so I cranked up the cardio. Yes. As the fat melts off, and your hormones become calibrated, the walking will become too easy. You are now in better physical condition and fitness level than you were a few months ago, so, you hit a plateau because there's not enough physical challenge. This is when you switch to inclined walking, or running, or boot camp classes. Something that is more physically challenging than the walking.

Like any exercise program, as you adapt, you have to intensify it.™

Also, I need to point out that at the beginning, you are not going to see your fat come off. What! Yes, that's right. In the beginning you will not see the fat coming off. If you've been gaining weight month after month, year after year, your cells are sugarcoated.

Yes, your cells are SUGARCOATED.™

This is known to the diabetic as the Hemoglobin A1c test. It is a test to see how much sugar is coating the hemoglobin within your red blood cells. If you are overweight and gaining, your entire body is sugarcoated, and your bloodstream is packed with sugar. Therefore, in the beginning as you cut calories, your body is not going to metabolize the body fat. It's going to start with burning off the sugarcoating in-and-around your cells.

Most people who lose 50-75-100 pounds will attest to this fact. They will say, "In the beginning the fat came off very slowly, and then after a few months it just started melting off."

The fat "Melt Off" occurs when your body has cleaned out and used up all of the sugarcoating.

The reverse of this process occurs when you go from your ideal weight to being overweight. If you are at your ideal weight, you can overeat for several weeks and not gain much fat. Why? Because a lot of the excess calories are being stored as "Sugar Coating", and not as body fat.

Then, if you keep overeating, one day, you notice that, "Everything I eat turns to fat." This stage occurs because your body is completely sugarcoated and packed with sugar, and so any excess calories that are not immediately burned will turn into body fat.

So now you are back at square one again, where you start cutting back on your caloric intake and the fat doesn't come off right away because your body is burning off the sugarcoating. Once that's done, then it will go after the body fat exclusively, hence, the melt-off stage.

So the "cupcake" diet that this doctor is selling and to everyone who is looking for a shortcut, I've got a news flash for you. There is no shortcut. Just like the teenage scientists who put their teacher on a calorie-controlled diet of 2000 calories a day and he was able to lose 39 lbs in 90 days, the principle of fat loss, or muscle gain, or weight maintenance, is mostly math.

Your answer is in taking control of the numbers you're eating.™

Bodybuilders who can't gain muscle simply need to increase their calories. You work out and eat a little extra calories than you need. Then you should grow a little in size every week. If you work out heavier and hit every muscle group, eat more excess calories, you'll grow bigger still. When you get close to your goal weight, say 185 lbs for a 5'10" male, then you continue to work out but switch to maintenance calories. Gradually, any added fat that you gained while you were bulking up will be transformed into muscle in this phase. The key is to be sure you are consistently working out, and eating muscle-building meals. A double cheeseburger, large fries, and a milk shake will bulk you up, but with a lot more fat than muscle. And then you likely won't be able to lose that extra fat if you haven't invested the time to learn how to eat and make meals for yourself, and you end up being overweight for much of your life.

If you are already overweight, then work out and use your body fat for energy, don't consume excess calories or you'll wind up with a sumo-wrestler body.

Weight gain and weight loss is not something to be taken casually. Fat loss is tricky. Your body will resist you and your cravings for food will overcome you if you haven't got a solid knowledge-based mathematical plan.

I feel I've done that with the Number Crunch Diet™. And yes I do realize that many people lose weight on a wide range of other plans, but many people do not. Or they do and then they don't, i.e., they yo-yo. Imagine having flat lower abs in your fifties. You can be active with your kids, keep that bond with your spouse, and feel younger than your age. That's more likely to happen when food is no longer on your mind, and when you know exactly how much you can have of this or that, based on the fact that you know the calories and you know your body's requirement.

Your doctor may wonder what you are doing to be so fit when the majority of his patients are defined as being overweight. Tell him about the Number Crunch Diet™ and its Pre-Counted Meals™. Doctors get very little or no educational training in diet and nutrition during med-school. This is why people who enter med-school with an interest in health drop out of med-school, because they come to discover, med-school has very little to teach people about health. Don't be fooled by credentials and titles. And don't be fooled by the "cupcake diets".

CHAPTER 57

Crunch Time!

So now that you've got your feet wet, let's crunch the numbers on a food label!

Okay, so your eyes see hundreds of different foods, but your body only sees three foods. What are they? Protein Carbohydrate and Fat. Yes, it sees sugar, yes it sees fiber, cholesterol, sodium, vitamins, etc., but as far as Calories, there are only three foods.

So let's take ketchup. What kind of food does your body see when you give it ketchup? Carbohydrate. Yes, sodium, yes lycopene red color pigment, but ketchup is a nonfat nonprotein 100% carbohydrate food.

The label reads:
1T – measuring Tablespoon
17g – grams
servings per container about 40
the container is 24oz 680g, given on the front label at the bottom
E = 15   E energy = 15 calories
Cals from Fat = 0   as expected
Total Fat = 0g
Sat Fat = 0g   no fat, no saturated fat, makes sense
Trans Fat = 0g   no toxic poison fat, TF should always be zero
Chol = 0mg   no cholesterol, because it's found in animal products
Na = 150mg   150 milligrams of sodium as we expect in ketchup

CHO = 3g   3 grams of carbohydrate, times 4 = 12 calories
f = 0g   no fiber, tomatoes have fiber, ketchup does not
s = 2g   2 grams of sugar carbs, times 4 = 8 calories of sugar
Prot = 0g   no protein, as expected

Notice that I converted carbs to calories by multiplying by 4. Recall our NCD rule, "Weigh in Grams, Crunch in Calories".

So of our three foods, fat carbs prot, our calories are 0 12 0, adding them together = 12 total calories per 1T 17g serving of ketchup.

Do you see a discrepancy? The E energy calories at the top says it is 15 calories per 1T 17g serving, but we calculated 12. That's just the way it goes sometimes. Not all food labels will match up exactly.

Let's try dry powdered milk. What kind of food is dry milk? Well, it's nonfat, it's milk carbs and milk protein.
The Nutrition Facts state:
1/3cup 23g
80 servings per box
the box is 4lbs 64oz 1.81Kg 1810g (kilograms times 1000 = g)
E = 80 calories
F = 0
SF = 0
TF = 0
Polyunsat Fat = 0
Monounsat Fat = 0
Chol <5mg (the < symbol looks like an "L", for Less-than)
Na = 125mg
K = 390mg   K=potassium, this is a high potassium food
CHO = 12g   carbs=12g x4 = 48 calories
f = 0
s = 12g   sugar calories are 12x4=48cals
Prot = 8g   protein calories are 8g x4 = 32 calories

There's no fat, as expected, and therefore, no saturated fat, no polyunsaturated fat, which we don't pay attention to, no monounsaturated fat, which we call omega-9, again, not going to pay attention to this. No TF, always check the label for this and never buy anything that has a number there other than zero. "No" cholesterol, less-than 5mg. Some sodium, 125mg. Significant potassium, that's good, because potassium is needed to balance out the sodium in our diet, and is found naturally in fruits and vegetables, and dry milk. So our glass of NF milk is like getting a serving of potassium from one large apple. Carbs, we converted grams to calories, and got 48. Fiber, dairy products have no fiber. Sugar, all the carbs are sugar carbs, lactose, milk sugar. Protein, converted into calories = 32.

Did you see all that?

Now let's go further. What is the total calories of fat + carbs + protein? It's 0 + 48 + 32 = 80 calories. This matches the E energy calories at the top, 80. So this is an example where the food label is exactly accurate in this regard.

Let's do 2% milk.
What do we know about 2% milk? In terms of our three foods? Well, it's low-fat milk, so in addition to milk sugar and milk protein, it's got some milk fat.

The label reads:
1cup 240 mL
servings 16   it's a gallon of milk, 3.78L liters, 3780mL milli Liters
E = 130 calories
F = 45 cals
total fat = 5g   to convert to cals, times 9, 5x9=45 calories of fat
SF = 3g   times 9 = 27 calories of saturated fat
TF = 0g   always zero, per NCD rules
Chol = 25mg   animal fat is where we get dietary cholesterol from
Na = 130mg   not a high sodium food
CHO = 13g   times 4 = 52 calories of carbohydrate
f = 0g
s = 13g = 52 calories
Prot = 10g   times 4 = 40cals

So, with regard to our three foods, what's the total calories? Fat = 45, Carbs = 52, Prot = 40, 45+52+40=137 calories. The E was 130 calories at the top, so it's close, and it will have to do. Just be aware that the numbers won't match exactly with all foods, as it did with the dry milk, 80 and 80.

Okay, let's go deeper with the numbers.

We have three things that make up the whole, what are they again? Fat CHO Prot. What is the whole? E or calories, energy. Why is this important? Because if we are taking in more energy than we need, the body stores that extra energy, either as adipose tissue (visible body fat), or glycogen (invisible muscle storage energy), or glycation (cellular sugarcoating).

Note, if you are lean and at your ideal weight, the storing of excess energy as glycogen is a good thing, as this energy will be there for your workout the next day, allowing you to achieve a good hard workout. This is the principle of "Carb-Load" and FFS. Just be sure you really do work out. If you carb-load and don't work out, then eventually that will catch up with you and your carb-loading will turn into visible body fat.

So our three parts of the whole are, fats carbs protein. Think of one dollar in money, and that you have nickels dimes and quarters. Two quarters, four dimes, and two nickels = $1.00. One quarter, 6 dimes, and 3 nickels = $1.00. Three quarters, 2 dimes, and 1 nickel = $1.00. The three always equal the whole. Same is true for protein carbohydrate and fat. They add up to the total calories.

If I have $1.00 total and I have 4 dimes, what percent of my money is dimes? $0.40 over $1.00 or 40/100 = 0.4 times 100 = 40%. If I have a total of $1.00 and I have one quarter, what percent of my money is the quarter? $0.25 divided by $1.00 or 25/100 = 0.25 times 100 = 25%.

If I have 45 calories of fat, and the total calories are 137 calories, what percent of my calories are from fat? 45/137 x 100 = 33%.

If I have 52 calories of carbs and 137 total calories, what percent of my calories are from carbs? 52/137 x100 = 38%.

If I have 40 calories of protein and 137 total calories, what percent of my calories are from protein? 40/137 x100 = 29%.

So our glass of 2% milk is 38% carbs 33% fat and 29% protein. This is very close to 40 30 30, the NCD target. So, 2% milk is actually a macro-balanced food. The macronutrient percents, percent macros, "macros", is sort of "a third a third a third", or moderate carbs moderate fat moderate protein.

In fact, if ever I am somewhere and I need a meal, I stop at an AM/PM and buy a quart of 2% milk. Of all the available foods, 2% milk is the closest to being 40% carbs 30% fat 30% protein, it's 38 33 29.

This is my advice to you as well. Skip all of the other options, and drink a quart of 2% milk, chugging down say 16oz to satisfy your immediate hunger, and then finish the remaining 16oz gradually. The E is 130 calories per 8oz cup, so, times 4 cups per quart = 520 calories. One quart of 2% milk is a ~500 calorie meal.

The NCD Emergency Meal™ ONE QUART OF 2% MILK

But you say, "I can't drink milk." Well, buy good-quality milk. It is true, not all milk is the same. I pay $14.99 per gallon for raw milk at the healthfood store. This is five times the price of regular milk, but it's also five times better for you.

Raw milk, if you live in California, is legal. Although "they" have tried to outlaw it and put this farmer out of business. Shame shame big business and government. My mother drank raw milk. Your ancestors drank raw milk. A goat or a cow were valuable possessions in Biblical times, and throughout history.

Raw milk is unpasteurized, therefore, not heated, the proteins are alive. Raw milk is not homogenized, meaning, it's not spun at a high speed to break up the milk fat into tiny lipid bullets. Yes bullets. There are researchers that believe that the homogenization of milk, the centrifugation of the milk, spinning it at a high speed, to break up the milk fat, i.e., homogenize it, is a cause of blood vessel wall inflammation and arterial plaque buildup.

These tiny lipid bullets are damaging the walls of the endothelial lining, causing them to inflame, and then your body's response is to patch it with cholesterol and calcium to prevent internal bleeding. Your body compensated to allow you to survive. But with narrowing of the inside of your blood vessel. But at least you're alive. You can do your own research on the subject. Just choose Raw Milk over Pasteurized Homogenized (heated and spun) Milk. Your ancestors, and your ancestor's ancestors, didn't pasteurize and homogenize their milk.

Raw milk is also your first choice for…PROBIOTICS! Yes, we hear so much about probiotics, our normal gut flora, good bacteria. Yogurt is fine, but yoghurt and kefir and other dairy sources of probiotics are nowhere near as effective at establishing good normal colon function as raw milk. If you have any kind of colon disorder or gastrointestinal problems, in my opinion, raw milk will fix it. This is why I pay $15 a gallon for milk. It's my healthy gastrointestinal insurance plan.

If you live in a state that outlaws raw milk. How stupid is that. Outlaws raw milk. A food that has been consumed for centuries, and is still consumed by people in underdeveloped nations. These "poor" people are drinking the most expensive milk on the planet, and without their government telling them that they can't. So, you can push for legislative freedom to drink raw milk, or you can contact your local dairy farmer, whose family drinks raw milk, and see if you can buy a portion of a cow. As co-owner of the cow, you are free to drink its milk raw. If you are a dairy farmer, you might look into marketing this to expand your business.

The raw milk dairy that I purchase milk from is called Organic Pastures, and you can read about the safety and health benefits of raw milk at their website www.organicpastures.com. They even have an annual "Camping with the Cows" customer appreciation event, where you can take your kids and a tent and sleep outdoors, learn about organic farming, and take part in the quart-of-milk-chugging contest. How fun is that!! I betcha I could win! So support your local raw milk farmers.

The NCD says GOOD milk is GOOD food.™

If you are lactose intolerant, you likely just have bad gut flora. Drink raw milk or take probiotics to colonize your colon with good bacteria. Try drinking sterile milk. It's in the grocery aisle, aka, UHT milk, ultra high temperature milk. It's more expensive, but chances are it's the bad bacteria in the cheap milk that you are intolerant to, not the milk sugar. If your mother gave you milk as an infant, which every newborn baby had, then you had the lactase enzyme when you were born. Your DNA worked then. If your DNA worked then, why wouldn't it work today? The lactose-intolerant campaign is, in my opinion, just a way to sell more varieties of products, from soy milk, to almond milk, to lactose-free milk. It's like the six-different varieties of fancy fish oils when you only need one, the original one.

If you are intolerant to milk, you can make your own UHT milk to save money. Take one gallon of 2% milk and fill eight of your 20oz Sobe beverage bottles with 16oz of milk, the line just below the word "Sobe" is the 16oz mark. Place them in the microwave in a ring/circle. Turn the microwave plate and adjust the bottles so that all the bottles are touching one another and your circle of bottles is centered on the plate. Press 15 minutes and high. If your microwave is less-than 1200 watts you will have to add more time. At the end of 15 minutes, use a thermometer to check the milk's temperature. Sterilization requires two seconds at 132°F. Check all eight bottles to see that the temperature needle rises above 130 and slows down and stops before 140. Take your readings quickly as the temperatures are dropping from the moment the microwave stops. If your needle stops at 120°F, then that bottle needs another 30 seconds in the microwave. If your needle goes above 140°F, you may need to cut back on the sterilization time, and also be sure to fill all of your bottles evenly to the same 16oz level, and be sure your circle of bottles is centered on the plate and that the bottles were touching one another and in a true circle. Once you've made a few batches correctly, you can omit the temperature-taking step as you've got the procedure mastered. The final step (optional), is to top each bottle off with 4oz of water to bring the volume up to 20oz, one full Sobe bottle, with an inch of air at the top. Cap the bottles, let cool, and refrigerate. You just made UHT milk for 1/5th of the supermarket price. Pretty cool huh.

The NCD Milk Sterilization™ procedure

I made this sterile milk when I first started drinking milk as I was reacting to dairy. Clearly I am talking from experience. I fixed my intolerance to milk, and began drinking one quart a day religiously, and still do today.

The NCD recommends that you wean yourself back on to milk.™

After about a year of drinking two gallons of sterile 2% milk per week, I was able to switch to unsterilized regular good-quality milk. Then when Lassen's opened up, I switched to raw milk. The milk naysayer people simply haven't troubleshot their problem by drinking sterile milk. The raw-milk naysayer people are simply ignorant of history and nutrition, or part of an agenda to remove raw milk from the market. My advice is solid. I went from "lactose intolerant" to drinking dozens of gallons of "dangerous" raw milk each year. I knew my DNA could make lactase. And I'll bet yours can too.

The NCD Lactose Intolerance™ protocol
1. Wean yourself back on to milk. Begin with sterile 2% milk. Start with 2oz every-other-day, then 2oz every day. Then increase it to 4oz a day, then 4oz twice a day. Then 8oz a day, and then 8oz twice a day every-other-day, and then 8oz twice-a-day every day. Then 16oz a day. Then 16oz twice a day every-other-day. Then 16oz twice a day = one quart a day. Timeframe, 4-6 weeks.

2. Then try a good-quality regular 2% milk.
3. Then switch to 2% raw milk (50/50 whole milk and nonfat).

While traveling in July through Arizona on a trip to the Grand Canyon, I found a bottle of my sterile milk in a bag in the trunk of the car. If you've ever been to the Grand Canyon in July, then I don't need to tell you how hot the bottle was at 3pm in the afternoon. I wondered if it was okay to drink, so I opened it and it was perfectly fine. I drank it and no problem. It had been sterilized so there were no living bacteria to cause the milk to spoil. This is the reason UHT milk in the grocery aisle has a 6-8 month expiration date at room temperature, it's sterile. So for the lactose-intolerant people out there, take another look at your problem.

You shouldn't be intolerant of anything. Whether it be milk, egg whites, peanuts, strawberries, or people. A healthy person doesn't let things "get to them". You tolerate it. It doesn't get to you. It doesn't affect you. The food, or the person, can't make you react. I can control my television set using the remote control. I press the button, and the TV responds. For some of you, I just described your relationship with other people. The reason for your stress. It's fine to "not be a fan" of certain foods, but not when it comes to milk. Yes, there are some people of Asian descent that can't make the lactase enzyme, but they are a small percentage of the population, not 40-million Americans, or 33-60 percent of this group and that group. If you made lactase when you were born, then you can make it now. You may just have to wake up that part of your DNA, and begin doing so by drinking sterilized 2% milk, because your real intolerance is to the bad bacteria, or pus, found in cheap milk.

So keep a quart of UHT 2% milk in your car for those times when you've gone more than four hours without eating. It's a good source of nutrition, it has close to 30% protein to sustain you and satisfy your hunger, the fat and carbs make it taste delicious, the party part, and it's 500 total calories, a meal, the NCD Emergency Meal™. Or for a 250-calorie snack, have 16 ounces, the Sobe bottle, the NCD Sterile Milk™.

CHAPTER 58

The Wrap-up

So did ya have fun! I did. I could give you more "Selfcare Strategies" but there comes a point when it's time to put the book down and put what you've learned into ACTION!

Action is what makes it happen. Knowledge + Action = Results

My suggestion is to start with one TCY recipe, say the NCD Hard Shell Tacos™, read it, make a list of the things you need to make it, then pick a day when you have time, and make it. Be sure to not deviate from the recipe or you will not end up with 500-calorie meals that are 40% carbs 30% fat 30% protein.

Well, some of you may say, this is too high carb for my body type, or it's too much protein. I recommend you read the very well-known book, written by Barry Sears PhD, called *The Zone*. I was working with a lab assistant and she had taken the book out from the library and brought it to work to read but it was a bit over her head. I was reading another book at the time, so I wasn't all that interested in her book. She kept telling me that she couldn't figure out why she kept bringing the book to work when she knew she wasn't going to read it. Then I picked the book up and that book changed my life. God kept having her bring that book to work because He wanted Me to read it.

My hope for you is that you recognize a good thing when you see it and that you realize that it's no accident that you have read this book. It is my sincere hope that the ABC Water™ and the Number Crunch Diet™ will improve your life as much as they have improved mine.

To summarize everything discussed would take another 50 pages, instead, I suggest you go back and read it from the beginning as it really is an action plan like no other out there.

Bridging The Reader From Advice To Results – JPM™

The principles of the ABC Water™ may be simplified into one phrase. Target your urine pH to be at exactly 7. Or 6.5 if you like.

The Number Crunch Diet™ premise is, you eat 500 calories per meal, comprised of 40% carbohydrate 30% fat and 30% protein, thereby making calorie counting easy by consuming Pre-Counted Number Crunched Meals™.

The best way to make them a part of your life is to just start doing them. Like everything in life, it will become clearer with practice.

Thank you for purchasing and reading my book. If it's benefited you, return the favor and send someone to the website. I believe that acid-base balance and weight control can potentially fix 80% of all the health problems out there.

CHAPTER 59

SUMMARY INDEX

This chapter includes a list of ORIGINAL phrases, sayings, or statements that I the author personally coined. So, if you see anything from this list being used elsewhere, if their intention is to bring readers to my book and they cite it, then thank them. If you see anything from this list being used elsewhere and the person, writer, or website is appearing as though they are the original author, they are not. They have taken it, from this publication.

ABC Water™

a step by step solution to ALKALINE DEFICIENCY™

the Number Crunch Diet™

count calories by counting Pre-Counted Meals™

12 Changes a Year™

Build a NCD Recipe Repertoire™

Jumper Publications & Media™

A jumper is a device that connects one wire on a circuit board to another, allowing for, the transfer of information from one to the other.™

JPM and the author make no claims that the reader will experience any of the benefits stated in this book from drinking ABC Water or the Number Crunch Diet.™

Any decision to implement a lifestyle or dietary change based on information in this book is 100% the reader's own choice. We simply show you how it can be done, step by step, in full detail.™

JPM and the author are not liable for any harm or damages arising from the contents of its publications. Reading beyond the Introduction is the reader's consent and agreement to this disclaimer and release of any and all liability.™

ABC stands for Alkaline, vitamin B, vitamin C.™

When I felt fatigued, my urine pH was 5.™

The fatigue from physical activity is in part due to the acid, and the sooner you mop it up, the better you will feel.™

And the number-one thing you or I or anyone else should be doing is, keeping your body pH slightly alkaline and avoid becoming acidic.™

Make the ABC Water according to the recipe formulation and notice the change in how you feel when you bump your urine pH up from 5 to 6 to 7.™

My alkaline consumption, from dietary fruits and vegetables, is not sufficient for my acid production, from dietary protein and physical exercise. I need to supplement.™

I cannot say anything about you personally, because I do not know you personally. I can only tell you what I do, and what I can reasonably generalize about others.™

Mental stress is the worst type of all acid-producers, because it doesn't stop.™

Replaying mental stress over-and-over in your head produces a never-ending 24/7 supply of acid.™

You don't want to tap into your alkaline stores if you don't need to.™

You need all the B vitamins, in a steady stream, rather than a once-a-day dose.™

If you plan on drinking ABC Water every day like I do, then you'll want the purest supplements on the market, otherwise, you could be potentially doing more harm than good by exposing yourself to a daily dose of trace contaminants.™

Each person has to determine for themselves how much alkaline supplementation is needed to keep your body alkaline and to prevent tapping into your alkaline reserves.™

If you run deficient on a daily basis, then eventually you'll use up all your alkaline stores.™

A healthy 20-year-old vegetarian who doesn't work out hard likely doesn't need any additional alkalinity. It is up to the reader to determine his or her alkaline status.™

Vitamin C is your body's primary water-soluble antioxidant, combatting the aging effects of free-radical damage, or, "rust".™

You need vitamin C daily, and a steady supply is best.™

ABC Water Formulation™
2.5t   sodium bicarbonate
2.5t   potassium bicarbonate
1cap   vitamin B complex
1/2t   vitamin C powder
1 gallon reverse-osmosis water or good-quality water

Soft plastics leach, water is a dissolver, it likes to pick up things.™

You have to think about everything you do. Are you doing it by your own choice? Or because of repeat advertising?™

Plastic chemicals disrupt the body's hormonal system.™

Rather than worry about the number on the bottom of the container, just use glass.™

But worse than microorganisms are, Chemicals.™

Chlorine used to purify the drinking-water can cause endothelial linings to inflame and your body's response is to thicken them.™

Both distilled water and reverse-osmosis water lack minerals, so I supplement.™

Getting people to believe that plastic-bottled water is better than tap water or filtered-tap water is the same as when they told us that margarine was better than butter and good for your heart, when in fact the world has been told that margarine is the most toxic fat in the supermarket.™

Go Green with Glass!™

Eating homemade food is the key to maintaining proper weight and good health.™

The purpose of your refrigerator is to store the energy and nutrition you need to live your life.™

If you fill your SKS glass container to the brim, then screw on the cap, your meals can last 10-14 days without spoiling!™

If your coworkers judge you by the labels on your clothes, then show up with a glass water bottle and glass straw and see who has more class, and more smarts.™

The ABC Water Glass Beverage Container.™

Top-of-the-list, number one thing that I consider of prime health importance is stocking up your alkaline reserves and keeping them stocked.™

Since a vegan diet is not an option for many of us, myself included, the next best thing you can do is to supplement with bicarbonate. But before you do so, you need to determine your current alkaline status to see where you're at.™

Show the world how classy you are and how informed and cutting-edge you are by drinking your beverage from a glass container and using a $9 glass straw.™

It could be that if you balance your acid alkaline status all your symptoms might go away.™

Rather than treat the problem, fix your health status, and the problem goes away as a byproduct of having good health.™

A normal healthy body should have a balance of acid neutralization going on in the body, and this gets reflected in the urine.™

If you don't have enough alkaline reserves, then your body is going to hold on to any and all alkaline that you have and your urine is going to be excreted as an acid, pH 5or 6.™

Just because something is COMMON, that doesn't make it NORMAL.™

You want your body to have a sufficient account balance of alkalinity. NSF, no sufficient funds, is not healthy.™

A lot of things in life are, which came first, the chicken or the egg?

An alkaline diet, the vegan vegetarian diet, is the best way to keep the acid from becoming a problem.™

Is it any wonder people are sick? The scales are tipped to the wrong side.™

But there is a workaround solution for those of us who aren't vegetarians or eat few fruits and vegetables, you can supplement with bicarbonate. But you have to do it sensibly and responsibly.™

With dieting, you want to track your calories, with alkalinity, you want to track your urine pH.™

Before you begin drinking the ABC Water, you will test the pH of all of your urinations for one week to see "where you're at".™

You want to become familiar with your urine-pH numbers.™

The most telling urine-pH number is the one when you first get up, never miss testing this one.™

The goal is to have all of your urinations be exactly 7. Not less-than 7, not greater-than 7.™

You don't want to overshoot, so if you get a 7.2, no more ABC Water for the rest of the day, if you get a 7.4, no more ABC Water for 24 hours or longer. Your target is 7 exactly.™

Be on the lookout for when your body's alkaline stores become stocked up and at that point you then switch from Stocking-Up Mode to Maintenance Mode.™

Checking the status of the internal environment of your body, the "vehicle" that makes or breaks your life, should be of paramount importance to you.™

This is not a medical book for medical problems, it's a selfcare book for optimum health.™

We discard our urine down the bowl, never realizing that this liquid just left our kidneys, which just left our blood, which just circulated throughout our entire body.™

The first sign of liver damage, as a result of taking certain things that are "hard on the liver", is a change in urine color from yellow to amber that persists despite hydration and a changing diet.™

Just touch the edge of the paper to the liquid and pull away. Don't Dip! The liquid will travel up the paper.™

Later, I decided to have 4-6oz of ABC Water one-hour before bed to ensure that my body had some alkalinity available to mop up the acid created during sleep.™

I also noticed that when I did consume plenty of fruits and vegetables, that it did raise my pH, so it's true, an alkaline diet is a diet high in fruits and vegetables, and this should be everyone's first choice for alkalinity.™

And yet, it's the foundation of health, the pH acid-alkaline status of your internal environment.™

Could the ADHD kids simply be experiencing the physiology of acidosis?™

Because bicarbonate is alkaline, you don't want to drink it 30 minutes before a meal or within 2 hours after a meal.™

Like anything you eat or drink, you should be in a calm and relaxed state, no multitasking.™

The ABC Water is meant to be sipped GRADUALLY throughout the day.™

Don't be shy, tell people what you are drinking and refer them to where they can purchase a copy of this book.™

Tell them about Jumper Publications, and the Selfcare Strategies.™

ABC Water can fill in the gap where your fruits and vegetables aren't quite cutting it.™

The five general categories that a person might see.™
1. The Ammonia Smell
2. The Highly Acidic
3. The Moderately Acid
4. The Slightly Acid
5. The Healthy Vegetarian

The Up Down Situation.™

My tissues were alkaline depleted, so any ABC Water that I consumed only made my urine briefly alkaline, as the bulk of the bicarbonate was being soaked up by my cells and tissues.™

I think there are people out there, agencies, that are aware that many people are alkaline deficient.™

Healthy newborn babies, who enter the world perfectly created, they also have a urine pH of 7.™

Not only does a Clinical Laboratory Scientist see and understand the patient's test results, they produced them!™

A steady diet of starches creates a soft-muscle body.™

Some people who are ill or have a health crisis turn to a 100% plant diet in an attempt to heal themselves, to fix their acid-base balance.™

There is the mixed approach, eat more fruits and vegetables, and supplement with bicarbonate every other day, but this is entirely an individual approach that only the reader can design for themselves.™

The vegan diet is essentially a diet whereby you carb-load every single day of your life.™

When you eat sugar with fat, as in desserts, the sugar raises insulin and the whole thing gets converted into body fat!™

NCD Fat Free Sunday™
NCD Half-day Fat Free Sunday™

The vegan diet is ideal for cleansing and detoxification due to its high alkalinity, plant fiber, living enzymes, and color pigments.™

Vitamin B is your energy vitamin, it's also anti-stress, so if you need a pick-me-up, instead of caffeine, try a little vitamin B, try the ABC Water.™

Vitamin C is responsible for Damage Control, fixing everything and trying to revert tissues and cells back to new again.™

NCD Hawaiian Pizza™

Ascorbic acid converts to Ascorbate in the presence of bicarbonate, and Ascorbate can go directly to the adrenal glands for stress reduction, this would make Ascorbate a Cortisol Crusher!™

"ANABOLIC" ASCORBATE™

For an added fatigue fighter, have 2oz of chicken breast before bed, a half hour after your 4-6oz of ABC Water, to provide your body with the amino acids it needs for body repair.™

With regard to your body's internal environment, and getting to know it by testing your urine pH, no doctor can do this for you.™

Taking control of your alkaline status is no different than taking control of your weight or finances, if it's to be, it's up to me.™

Remember, your goal is to simply use the ABC Water to bump your urine pH up to 7. If it's already at 7, then you don't need any additional alkalinity.™

Wouldn't it be nice if we could track our vitamin C or magnesium levels? Fortunately, we do have a way of tracking our body's acid alkaline status.™

In order to see patterns and to make correlations between how you feel and your urine pH, you will need to test and record all of your urinations for several weeks.™

Make notations or keep a journal, include things like, exercise, times when you were upset, high-protein dinners, high fruit-and-vegetable days. The more you put into it, the more likely it is that you will see patterns and relationships with your urine pH.™

Achy joints, hands, feet, muscles, back, that's often excess acid that hasn't been mopped up.™

Exercising when your body's already acidic is dangerous.™

If you already have acid or fatigue, and you work out again, you add acid on top of acid. When what you should be doing is recovering; hydration, nutrition, sleep, light-movement exercise, and alkalization.™

What people commonly do is mask their acidic state with caffeine, and Zoom Zoom, off they go!™

Think of a dart board, you want to keep landing your dart in the center of the bull's eye, 7.™

When you absorb an offense, it now lives in you and it can activate your physiology without you even being aware of it.™

The author's personal conclusions with regard to alkalosis.™
1. Acidosis causes me to feel fatigue.
2. Alkalosis and a urine pH of 7 gives me almost endless energy.
3. Raising the pH of my urine to 7 lowered my blood pressure.
4. One foot in the grave begins with the depletion of my alkaline reserves.

The principle behind the Atkins diet is sound, cut carbs, and especially sugar, and the fat falls off. The problem is, that at a certain point you become carb-depleted, and then one day you blow it and start eating all the carbs you had been depriving yourself of, hence, the Yo-Yo Dieting phenomenon.™

Number Crunched Meals™

Fat Loss Is A Numbers Game.   When you take control of the numbers, you take control of your weight.™

Technically, we should all be taking the diabetic approach to eating, that is, moderate carbs, not high carbs not low carbs, moderate fat, not high fat not low fat, and moderate protein, not high protein not low protein.™

Since we need fat for cell membranes and steroid hormones, and we need protein for enzymatic reactions, cell structure, and muscle, and we need glucose for cellular energy and brain function, doesn't it make sense that we should be getting a balance of all three at each meal?™

The macros for the NCD are targeted at being 40% carbs, 30% fat, and 30% protein, almost a third a third a third, with a slight tip towards the carbs.™

The 40% protein "Body Builder's Diet" is out, as you can eat a 40% protein meal once or twice a day, but not five times a day every day.™

To achieve fuller muscles or gain weight, you can tweak the percents to 50% carbs 25% fat 25% prot, NCD One Fruit 'Meal'.™

To cut fat, you can tweak the percents to 35% carbs 35% fat 30% protein, or even 30% carbs 40% fat and 30% protein, (see TCY).™

"Tweaking" as opposed to "Radical Shifts" is the preferred NCD approach due to the body's homeostatic mechanism to want to "Radically Shift Back to Where it Originally Was".™

You have to fool or trick your body so that it doesn't notice.™

Radical change is much harder to hold on to in the long term than gradual change.™

But what about the underlying symptoms? My theory is, that the person was already running on empty with regard to alkalinity.™

I believe, this compromise in acid-base balance in the body is the starting point for all other compromises that will follow.™

The real problem was below the surface, at the level of the fluids, that precious fluid that bathes the organs, the "Egg" if you will.™

Just keep eating, drinking, and doing all of those things that aren't good for you, it has nothing at all to do with this particular disease problem. Good grief.™

The problem is, there are people out there that had tumors and cancer and these ex-cancer patients are the ones making the claims that baking soda cured them.™

Keeping my blood slightly alkaline, and keeping my alkaline stores stocked up, for me is good insurance for cancer prevention, for me personally.™

Doctor Otto Warburg received a Nobel Prize for his discovery that cancer cannot survive in a high oxygen environment.™

Another way to get oxygen into the body is Cardiovascular Exercise. Sweat Cardio™

Get the tissues and the lymphatics and blood moving. Stagnant blood and lymph are like having stagnant bowels.™

The objective is to get your body to heal itself. What if you could skip all the treatment and just get your body to heal itself?™

No amount of Good will fix the Bad you are being exposed to on a daily basis.™

It's amazing what people Don't notice.™

The government has done its job and told us what causes cancer.™

Most people aren't doing much to identify the cancer-causing agents they are putting in their mouths, on their skin, in their lungs, into their tissues.™

NCD Taco Salad™

My beans weren't softening because my soaking-water was acidic and not alkaline. That's interesting.™

So the acid in the tomato juice hardens and the bicarbonate in the baking soda softens.™

What if high blood pressure is caused by the body being too acidic? What if, by alkalizing the body you could lower your blood pressure?™

That acidic blood makes vessel walls tighten, and that alkaline blood makes vessel walls soften, just makes sense to me.™

I'm surprised they don't call cancer "Essential Cancer".™

Don't let other people try to persuade you that something that's Abnormal is Normal.™

There being no treatment for getting rid of it, and you are told that you will take these pills for the rest of your life.™

Do you think God intended for us to have so many health problems, and hundreds-and-hundreds of disease names, more disease names every year?™

The "A" aspect of this book pertains to supplementing with alkalinity, due to a poor diet, physical exercise, and toxic stress. Even if you did eat 3-5 fruits and vegetables a day, you'd still likely come up short.™

ALAKALINE DEFICIENCY™

Isn't the founding principle of a "Free-Market Economy" that everyone gets to play?™

Think of calcium as having the same effect on your body as acidosis, tensing, and think of magnesium as doing the same thing as alkalizing, softening.™

NCD Beef Dip™

It would be nice if Lea & Perrins would DISCLOSE what exactly is in that "Natural Flavoring" they are using.™

Flavor should come from your food, not from chemical flavor enhancers.™

I would like to commend the Heinz corporation for revising their mustard label, which no longer lists "natural flavoring", but instead states five simple foods.™

Free sodium helps keep our body alkaline by grabbing precious bicarbonate from the urine and bringing it back into the body.™

So, sodium bicarbonate is a Double Alkalizer, as it dissociates into free sodium and free bicarbonate, both of which function to create alkalinity within the body.™

In backtracking to the root cause of hypertension and arterial plaque, the backtracking stops one or two steps short. This is done to prevent finger-pointing.™

There is no law that says anyone has to believe what the FDA says.

A vitamin is defined as a biological nutrient that we cannot make, and therefore we have to get it from our diets.™

Good sodium is free sodium, which can be obtained by eating plant foods, or can be supplemented by taking sodium-potassium bicarbonate when dietary intake is not enough.™

The thought occurred to me that the reason why I am eating so many Apricot Kernels and still want more is, maybe I'm low on vitamin B17!™

Unlike people who don't exercise, athletes and bodybuilders produce a lot of post-workout acid.™

The acid produced from exercise, if not neutralized and eliminated, can deplete alkaline stores. When this happens, your body "chokes".™

Exercise shouldn't take you to exhaustion, leaving "100% on the gym floor", as some fitness trainers advise.™

Instead of overeating to raise your energy, just alkalize.™

If your alkaline reserves are already depleted, you are at risk and in a dangerous physiological state.™

When what you should be doing is giving your body, Anti-Acid, Anti-Stress, and Anti-Oxidant, ABC Water, alkalinity, vitamin B, vitamin C, and hydration.™

A state of anabolism, (muscle growth), requires an alkaline internal environment, and your urine pH is the best indicator of this.™

The post-workout shake or meal is fine, but what really matters are the 6 to 12 to 18, 500-calorie meals you will be eating every 2.5-3 hours over the next 1-3 days during your growth and recovery period.™

Poor nutrition means poor recovery, poor muscle growth, and poor results, and then you give up, or worse, you turn to steroids to get some results.™

Your MEALS are FUELING your RECOVERY.™

Your post-workout shake is just one meal. What have you got planned and prepared in your refrigerator for your next 11 or 17 meals over the next 2 to 3 days?™

But what are you going to do in your 40s and 50s when your youth hormones are missing-in-action and you never took the time in your 20s and 30s to learn how to make your own meals and build a recipe repertoire?™

Don't be a cheater. Eat the Number Crunch Diet performance-enhancing meals instead.™

Along with the NCD meals used to speed recovery, try drinking the ABC Water and keeping your urine pH at 7 as a second way to speed recovery.™

Nip that acidosis in the bud, and get your body back to its healthy alkaline state ASAP. You'll feel better and have more energy.™

Another reason for keeping your urine pH at exactly 7 is for the prevention of crystals and stone formations, aka, renal calculi.™

The oxalates in tea bind to calcium in the blood or bones and show up in the urine as calcium oxalate crystals.™

Similarly, the phosphates in colas leach calcium out of the body. So pick your poison, colas or tea, you lose calcium either way.™

Alcohol dehydrates you causing your skin to age. Try to purge stress without alcohol, try the ABC Water.™

More than one ounce of wine at dinner means your motive has switched from enjoying dinner to getting a buzz and escaping your problems for a while.™

You never escape your problems or stresses. When the buzz wears off there will be your problems again, only now you're in a weaker state and less able to deal with them.™

The NCD doesn't allow "Moderation". Moderation is kind of middle-of-the-road, halfway there already. Instead, Rarely or Occasionally.™

You can fool your body into thinking it got caffeine by just having decaffeinated coffee. It's the placebo effect.™

A neutral urine pH of 7, (the same as plain water), is your safest bet to avoid crystals, and by abstaining from crystal-inducing beverages.™

There are many things that cause inflammation, but by keeping your urine pH at exactly 7, and not at 6, and definitely not at 5, you can, in my opinion, cross off one inflammatory factor from your list.™

The CHLORIDE is holding the sodium hostage in the bloodstream. Sodium is the good guy. It's the chloride that's bad.™

Less chloride means that sodium is free to leave the bloodstream and go do its job elsewhere in the body.™

They don't tell you the whole story.™

Your SYMPTOMS are SIGNS of COMPENSATION for something you are doing wrong.™

There are doctors going against the establishment and saying that, "Cholesterol has very little to do with increasing your risk of heart disease."™

These doctors then say that, "People are waking up to the truth."™

Someone once said, we dig our graves one mouthful at a time. There is wisdom in that. "Let food be thy medicine."™

You want to eat foods that supply free sodium, not sodium-chloride.™

So we have, refined white flour, refined white sugar, refined white salt. Choose God's design.™

MSG should never be consumed. The word "Flavoring" regardless of whether it says natural in front of it, can be just about anything, including MSG.™

"Spices" is another code word to be aware of.™

The biological harm of HFCS is well established so any food company that uses it in their products, is, in my opinion, untrustworthy.™

Do you find it interesting that there is so much public knowledge and talk about the heart, cancer, diabetes, lungs, thyroid, liver, pancreas, kidneys, gastrointestinal tract, gall bladder, brain, blood vessels, but no talk whatsoever about the INTERNAL STATE OF THE BODY.™

That the kidneys will change the pH of your urine to compensate for diet, therefore, if your urine is always acidic, your diet has excess acid byproducts, this is key.™

Come to find out, apple cider vinegar doesn't work to lower blood pressure in most cases, and the reason stated is that you have to alkalize the ACV with baking soda to get it to work.™

NCD Chicken Caesar Salad™

By keeping your urine pH at exactly 7 with the help of the ABC Water, you are artificially creating in your body the environment of a young healthy vegetarian.™

By keeping your urine at exactly 7 indicates that your body has neutralized excess acid.™

"An alkaline environment can be induced with sodium bicarbonate," or as in the case of the highly-perfected formula of the ABC Water, a combination of sodium-potassium bicarbonate.™

The body is producing acid, that's what it does, the problem occurs when the body's buffering systems are running on empty.™

The "bicarbonate" test result on your laboratory chemistry panel may be normal, however, this tells you little about the deficiency happening in the tissues and cells.™

Your blood levels are always going to be normal as long as there are supplies elsewhere in your body to draw from.™

By the time your blood work is abnormal, your body's supplies are already depleted.™

By the time your depletion shows up in the blood, you have a problem that's already rooted.™

If your doctor or anyone else says your urine pH is supposed to be acidic, wrong, as there are no normal values for urinary pH, as stated in the urinalysis textbooks.™

If the kidneys need bicarbonate to neutralize excess acid and it can't find any, where does it go next?   To the tissues, your pantry.™

Here's the key.   An acidic urine means there wasn't enough bicarbonate available so that the urine could leave the kidneys at a neutral pH of 7.   Alkaline Storage.   How does this happen?   Diet, Exercise, Stress.™

A urine pH of 5 is telling you about your internal alkaline reserves.™

If you are taking prescription medication you are under the care of your physician, this book is for the Selfcare Individual.™

Funny, we never hear about the #3 cause of death in America.™

Knowing the truth should empower you, so that as changes are occurring, you find yourself equipped with the "Tools" you need to navigate your way through the game of life.™

School books are one kind of information, the kind that everybody learns. Information Products are a completely different kind of information.™

Traditionally, Information Products have been for the select few, the elite, but now everyone has access to them.™

You can put yourself in that group of elite by reading what they read and knowing what they know.™

Much like how information about a particular company can give you an advantage in the stock market, so too can "Insider Information" about health, wellness, and disease.™

The kidney's second job after filtering the blood is to, reabsorb bicarbonate ions from the urine back-in to the kidney in order to maintain the blood pH at 7.4, aka, acid-base balance.™

Both doctors refused to use the words "alkaline" "alkalinity" "base" "acidosis" "acid" "pH" or "acid-base balance".™

Finally the nephrologist said, "They have diminished reserves." Diminished reserves of WHAT?™

Sadly, the average viewer of the program would not have caught all of the, what I will call as, mild-to-moderate deception for the sole purpose of winding up the program with a long list of supplements.™

Later on, the nephrologist said, "Something is putting them over the edge." But he wouldn't say what that "Something" is. You have in your hands a complete guide on how to personally take control of that "Something".

When the sand and debris have clogged the spray nozzle to the extent that you have only 15% of the water leaving the spray nozzle, you need a kidney transplant.™

Did the high pressure cause the kidney to fail? Or did the kidney damage cause the pressure to increase?™

The kidney, spray nozzle, gets damaged, and then the blood pressure goes up, in the garden hose. And then the two feed back on themselves compounding the problem.™

I am not bashing the medical system, it is doing exactly what it has been set up to do.™

It is the patient's job to find the answers, not the medical system's.™

When you fail to take Personal Responsibility in any area of your life, and it goes badly, you are the one to blame.™

They can tell you full truths, half truths, or no truths, it's their system.™

You have to SEEK the truth yourself to find the answers to your problems.™

If your urine pH is 5, then you are only a half a pH number away from having urine that's like white vinegar.™

So think of urine pH in terms of speed, 7 would be 70mph, 6 would be running on a treadmill, 5 would be a slow walk, and 4.5 the speed of a crawling baby, because the pH scale is logarithmic, every number is times ten.™

The NCD has a No Caffeine rule. Your goal is to get your body to have its own energy. Not to drug it into performing for you.™

Caffeine masks the underlying condition, that of acidosis.™

But what if you could raise your Zoom Zoom by raising your alkaline status?™

People with urine pHs of 5 and 4.5 are likely to be using caffeine for energy on a daily basis.™

Saying that your urine should be acidic is like the cardiologist in the 1980s telling his patients to use margarine.™

Fruit Test Sunday™

Aliquot – a number-crunched serving.™

Aliquoted – divided the whole into number-crunched servings.™

Aliquoting, the new term in dieting.™

NCD Sausage Pizza™

100 Calories Per Hour™

Boiling lean chicken breast to cook it removes most of the fat, resulting in NCD Fat Free Chicken.™

The NCD does not buy into the "Cheat Day" advice.™

Instead, one can do a FFS or HFFS carb-load using fresh in-season fruit. Pancakes with syrup or bread with jam are acceptable in the beginning until the desire for these foods wanes.™

JPM's methods are based on putting in effort to gain control and long-term results, leaving the cheating to the cheaters.™

You don't just eat carbs mindlessly.™

Carbs are like money, you have to earn them.™

You have to Earn your Carbs like you Earn your Money.™

On your FTS, after eating nothing but oranges, grapes, and watermelon, if your urine never hits 7, you're low on alkaline reserves.™

Your body's intelligence, in an attempt to save you, runs to the pantry for supplies and there's nothing there. The shelves have been emptied out.™

Lab tests check the blood levels, not the "pantry" levels.™

Then there's the slow drip, where month by month your "fluid" becomes a little darker.™

That they are combing the internet looking for anything that is a threat to the current way of thinking. Then they bash it. Who are they working for?™

And so it is with alkalosis, the subject rarely discussed in the mainstream, and yet, so important to good health, and its opposite, acidosis, playing a key role in so many ailments.™

After taking control of your alkaline status, the second-most important thing a person should do is take control of their weight by taking control of the numbers they're eating.™

The NCD will teach you to look at the meals and foods you are eating with greater insight and knowledge.™

When a nurse hangs an IV bag, she knows exactly what's in it and what it will do, similarly, you need to think of eating in this same manner.™

NCD Flaxseed Shakes™

Most diet plans differ in their macronutrient precents. The NCD is smack dab in the middle, nothing radical and no extremes.™

Just as correcting your Internal Environment can potentially have an effect of correcting a whole host of other health problems, so too it is with dropping excess body fat.™

Unique to the NCD recipes is a never-before-seen way of regularly eating Omega-3 fat, allowing for flexible cell membranes and softer skin.™

Since all NCD meals are 500 calories, tracking your intake becomes simple and easy with the NCD Pre-Counted Meals.™

You eat what you want and don't eat what you don't want.™

With some exceptions, no empty calories, no chemicals, no poisons, no stimulants. How do you expect to maintain a healthy weight if your bloodstream and tissues are short on nutrition, if food additives and artificial sweeteners are toying with your bodily functions, and inflammation and hormonal upset is being brought on by trans, burnt, and omega-6 fats and high-fructose corn syrup, food dyes and chemicals.™

Knowing the truth about what you are eating, you can't possibly continue eating it. You're Free.™

Chemical addiction isn't just for street drugs, it's for food too.™

By eating what you crave, you can, over time, eliminate your craving for it.™

With the NCD, you eat what you crave, and get it out of your system.™

EAT IT AND GET IT OUT OF YOUR SYSTEM™

Gradually, you will come to choose nutritious foods over treat foods and the treat foods will only be a small part of your diet.™

The one caveat is that your treat food has to be incorporated into a meal, and the NCD recipes help you to do this.™

With complete control of the numbers, you can work the NCD in any direction you want to go, weight loss, weight gain, or weight maintenance.™

If you crave ice cream, your body is asking for milk.™

If you crave ketchup, your body wants tomatoes.™

If you crave french fries, your body is looking for potatoes.™

See, when you become low on a nutrient, your body has you eating weird versions of that base food. This is the mechanism behind pica.™

Then, you overeat foods, trying to get the things you're missing in the foods you're eating.™

Your craving for ice cream can be eliminated by drinking milk.™

There are two yous. One that can drive your car across town. And the other that runs your internals, your Divine Intelligence.™

When it comes to deciding what to eat, the you that can drive your car across town needs to hand the steering wheel over to the inner you, and let your Divine Intelligence guide your food choices.™

You need to make all of your food choices from the inside, not from the outside, I want I want I want.™

Compensating is when you allow yourself to eat food because of a FEELING it will give you, doing something to mask something.™

If you find yourself eating for FEELING instead of listening to your Divine Intelligence, stop, catch yourself, be very aware of it. See it, and say to it, "Game Over, I know what you've been doing."™

When reading a book, tape additional blank pages to the back of the book so that when the new information mixes with your current information, you have a place to record your "Revelation Information".™

Revelations are your answers to becoming a better you.™

Everything on the ingredients label should be a food.™

If it's not a food, it's a chemical. A chemical addiction.™

NCD Ham & Pea Soup™

You have to make your own meals if you want to be successful at taking control of your weight by taking control of the numbers.™

Most restaurants tend to overcook the protein, rendering it semi-worthless, and even harmful.™

If you continually check with your Divine Intelligence when deciding what to eat, one day you'll ask it what it wants to eat and the response will be "Nothing Really". You are stocked up, nutritionally speaking.™

Stay full by not going more than four hours without eating.™

You don't lose fat by postponing meals. But rather, you put other people around you walking on thin ice.™

When cutting calories, never go below 80% of your maintenance requirement.™

Cutting calories by 30-40% is not going to fool your body's homeostatic mechanism, and then three-months later you'll be right back where you started.™

NCD KITCHEN CLOSED AT 5, 3-4-5 hours before bedtime will have you waking up thinner, and is an excellent way to lose fat.™

The NCD Calorie-Free Vegetables™ can be used to carry you to your next meal or to bedtime.

NCD Double Chew™ everything you eat to ensure proper digestion, absorption, and to slow down your eating, and thereby, decrease the amount you're eating.™

Put the Fork Down™ between mouthfuls of food.

NCD Pray Before Each Meal™, to draw a line between activities.

If your thyroid's become sluggish your lifestyle's become sluggish.™

Jumpstart a slow hypo thyroid with Sweat Cardio.™

Yeast thrive in an acidic environment of fermented food. If you're overweight with a sugar addiction, you need to raise your pH.™

For chronic yeast, all you may need to do is get that urine pH up from 5 to 6 to 7. Out of the fermentation zone.™

If you are in daily contact with things that have parasites, then you have parasites.™

You will never "unhook" yourself from a chemical food addiction as long as you keep eating it.™

To unhook yourself from a food item, try making a similar version yourself, so you can control the ingredients and use real foods, the NCD Quitting Plan.™

Weigh your ingredients instead of using measuring cups, it's more accurate and less dishes to wash.™

Whenever you see the words "Natural Flavoring" on a food label the NCD says to insert the phrase, "chemicals that make me addicted to their product".™

Chemicals work the same way regardless of where you put them.™

If you can, shop at the healthfood store, these companies list only real foods on their labels.™

Why is it that the average everyday supermarket has so many ingredients on their shelves that the consumer has no clue what they are?™

Every time you spend a dollar you vote.™

Imagine a shelf, reach forward and take a product off the shelf, now rotate it 180 degrees as you bring it towards you.™

NCD Food Craving Rules™
1. Eat the foods you crave and get them out of your system.
2. Don't eat chemicals or poisons, any word that is not a food.
3. Check with your Divine Intelligence as to what you are to eat.
4. Stay "full", never going more than four hours without eating.
5. To break addiction to a food, make something similar yourself.

"Calories In Calories Out" worked yesterday, today, and it will still work tomorrow, despite what the "experts" say on the cover of a magazine.™

I control the numbers, I control my size.™

The NCD Recalibration Exercise™ refers to cross-country-ski walking. Walking that Recalibrates Your Hormones.™

As you cut calories, your stomach shrinks, so some of your weight loss is simply from the clearing of your intestines.™

Teenage science students were successful at achieving fat loss through calorie counting, along with walking. The historical gold standard method.™

For those of you who are External, try letting your Internal control more of your decisions, understanding, and beliefs.™

No amount of Good can compensate for the Bad you continue to do. You have to eliminate the Bad.™

Sometimes, just Eliminating The Bad is all you need to do to feel better and get rid of your problem.™

If you are cutting calories you may find you need a bit of a boost. This can be done conservatively by using a small amount of 85% dark chocolate or 1oz of coffee with 3oz of whole milk. However, if you are on maintenance calories, you shouldn't be needing caffeine, or theobromine, caffeine's cousin found in cocoa.™

Caffeine is a drug, so treat it like a drug.™

Caffeine is cheating. It's energy without calories.™

Place the word Glycemic Load at the top of your list.™
Glycemic Load is the sugar-spiking capacity of your meal™

Insulin is your master hormone, if it ain't happy, none of your other hormones will be either.™

Move Cholesterol, HDL, LDL, to the bottom of your list, as they are merely distracting you from the important indicators, Insulin and Glycemic Load.™

When you wrap sugar and starch with protein, fat, and fiber, you slow down their insulin-spiking potential.™

You can also slow down the speed of the sugar by eating it gradually over 30-45-60 minutes, aka, infusion rate.™

Sugar has a function, so use it as needed, as the last thing you want is for your body to go into Famished Mode.™

NCD Roast Beef Sandwich™   NCD Chicken Bowl™

CarbFats, desserts, are allowed on the NCD but only as incorporated into a meal with 30% protein.

When I sit down to have a NCD meal, it's a party! And I party five times a day!™

Be A Role Model! I know you've got it in you! Live it!!

You will need to look for similar food items and sizes used in the recipes if you don't have the same supermarkets, so that the recipe tastes the same and so that the numbers are the same.™

Don't be caught without meals prepared and ready to eat.™

News Flash! There are no whole grains! What people think are whole grains are actually processed grains.™

The NCD is against "whole grains", but for sprouted grains.™

Forget about whole grains right here and right now.™

The NCD allows you to have 200 calories of carbs with each meal, the key is to pick-and-choose what carbohydrate food you want to eat, and don't eat carbs that you don't particularly want.™

Think about the amount of empty carb calories in one hamburger combo meal. Top and bottom bun, deep-fried potato starch, sugar ketchup, and a fountain drink. If this is you, Repent. And move forward this day to become a new healthier more productive you.™

Deep-fried oil is poison. Don't eat it. Your body has no use for oil that's been heated to 425 degrees.™

There are better ways to eat your food than to submerge it in oil at 425°F. You simply must put an end to this bad dietary habit.™

NCD Crackers Turkey Cheese™   NCD Salmon & Steak Fries™
NCD Pork Chop Mushroom Gravy Steak Fries™

Keep in mind that if you eat potatoes, such as baked potatoes or red potatoes, you won't have any desire for the adulterated versions.™

Eat the real thing and the craving for the processed version will fade away.™

The fat-loss industry is no different from the medical industry, in that, they partially help you, but they partially let you fail, so that they can fully keep your money.™

Don't even think about eating grains. Just when you want them, then have them. Otherwise, Just Say No To Grains.™

The NCD Buckwheat Oatmeal™ is a great alternative to wheat, as it is not a grain, but rather it's a fruit seed related to rhubarb.™

The carb and fat portions of your meal are your party parts. Pick and choose them wisely, asking yourself, "What do I want for carbs?"™

Whole grains, which are really processed grains, is an agenda to make and keep you fat. Then what happens?™

NCD Steak Bowl™   NCD Chicken Lasagna™

Weight Loss, Weight Gain, Weight Maintenance, is a Numbers Game, primarily.™

A moderate approach to weight loss is more likely to fool your body into shedding pounds without it noticing.™

The Number Crunch Diet is a food-additive chemical free diet, allowed only rarely to occasionally.™

The NCD is a diet whereby you make your own meals, as nutrition and calorie control are key principles of the program.™

Taste and Flavor are important, but they come third, as you are not eating for your external you, you are eating for your internal you.™

Just keep that refrigerator stocked with meals and use those meals to fuel your busy life, fitness goals, and longevity.™

The NCD is a low moody, no rollercoaster diet.™

In fact, don't be surprised if people around you begin to notice how calm, stable, and consistently productive you are.™

Pay attention to ingredients. Titanium is not a food.™

If you prefer to eat 1000-calorie meals, the NCD is flexible to this. Just have a double meal for breakfast, lunch meal plus a shake, and a double meal for dinner, 3000 calories. Just track your numbers.™

Have your lunch date at the park, save money and eat better, the NCD Picnic.™

NCD Four Bean Chicken Salad™

Do not count your intake in grams. This is just another way to make you fail. Energy is counted in calories. So convert grams to calories. Measure in Grams but Count in Calories.™

Aim for eating 80% of your food raw. When boiling vegetables or cooking proteins, cook it to 3/4ths doneness or MW and then allow it to OFF-HEAT COOK to just right.™

Do not overkill cook your proteins, or any cooked meals.™

If you stir-fry vegetables, do so in water, then toss them in oil off heat to protect the oil from heating.™

The NCD Fat Definitions™
Plant   Omega-9   Omega-6   Omega-3
'Animal'   Fish fat   Saturated fat

The NCD Edible Fats™
1. omega-9   olives, avocados, peanuts
2. omega-3   flax, chia, hemp
3. fish fat
4. animal fats and coconut oil

Refined corn, safflower, sunflower, and cottonseed oils are "Bad".

Forget the word "polyunsaturated" as it clumps good Omega-3 in with "bad" Omega-6, resulting in confusion.™

Fryer fat and Hydrogenated fat are NCD NonEdible Fats.™

Omega-6 foods yes, omega-6 refined oil no, NCD Omega-6 rule.™

Organic canola oil is fine for the NCD Garlic Green Beans.™
Soybean oil is fine in the NCD Coleslaw Dressing™
These fall under the Rare-to-Occasional rule. Just not daily, steady, or moderately.

Solvent extraction is common in nonorganic canola oil, so buy organic and look for the words "No Hexane" on the label.™

The Asian way of stir-frying in hot oil and the Western way of deep-frying food in hot oil are the same, both bad and outdated cooking methods that damage your health.™

Boiling in water pulls fat and impurities out of the food.™

Olive oil, avocados, and peanuts should be consumed Uncooked.™

Choose coconut oil for baking to cut down on using butter.™

Use butter on the NCD Popcorn and in the NCD Curry Sauce when the dish requires that nice buttery flavor.™

Many small-country farmers grow their food organically by default, that's all they know, so organic labeling is not necessary for them and allows for lower prices for their organic products.™

Clearly there are two types of food manufacturers, Good and Evil, high-technology chemicals and engineering versus old-fashioned traditional organic methods.™

Nuts are a mixture of fatty acid types, with walnuts being the oddball, high in omega-3.™

NCD Favorite Breakfast™

The NCD uses canned salmon instead of fresh or frozen salmon for three reasons.™
1. it's protected from light
2. it's protected from air
3. it's wild caught, not farm raised

Remember that the "U Shape" of the omega-3 and DHA EPA fatty acids makes them very unstable and quick to spoil.™

Fish and flax seeds need to be consumed or frozen on the day caught or ground, NCD Fresh Oil rule.™

Oils turn rancid by the oxidation from air and from light.™

Like the Cranberry, God made flax seeds with a specific purpose.

The NCD Essential Fats™   1. flax seeds
                           2. fish oil

Essential means we need to "seek them out" in our diet, eat them, consume them, NCD Dietary Essentials.™

Do you see how a diet high in fastfood, processed food, refined food, nutrient-depleted food, high-tech food, is going to be missing a lot of the Essentials?™

Health problems are due to a decades-long lack of Essential

Dietary Nutrients, lack of Good, and compounded with a steady flood of Bad, in my opinion.™

The NCD recipes include proteins from all sources, and including the NCD Forgotten Protein Meal™.

Phytonutrients (plant color pigments) should be at the top of your list when choosing foods.™

The NCD Six Color Groups™
White   Yellow   Orange   Red   Green   PBB

The NCD Leafy Greens™ protocol
week 1 Cilantro
week 2 Kale or Swiss Chard
week 3 Spinach
week 4 Spring Mix
NCD Wheat Grass Shot™ – if they didn't look fresh.

The NCD Four T Vegetable™ protocol
week 1 broccoli
week 2 brussel sprouts
week 3 cauliflower
week 4 coleslaw

NCD Color Vegetable™ protocol
1. cucumber (or organic zucchini)
2. bell pepper
3. carrots (and celery)
4. tomatoes
5. green beans
6. snap peas
7. beets

NCD Grapefruit™ free calorie 3oz "vegetable".

Any time you eat one of the above vegetables, give yourself a pat on the back, and for Beets, you get a pat on both sides!™

315

Be sure to check your supermarkets weekly for seasonal sales on fruits and vegetables to take advantage of the prices and get your fill of those nutrients until next year.™

NCD Orange Chicken™   NCD Lemonade™

Avoid the nine GMO crops, ACCC PSSSZ.™

Buy organic as much as possible, and this includes meat and dairy, since GMO feed is fed to nonorganic livestock. GMO is no different than margarine in the 1970s and 80s, adulteration of the food supply.™ Europe has a 'zero tolerance' for GMOs.

Sprinkle your food with a little Turmeric, Curry, or Cloves.™

NCD Orange Shake includes whey protein from food, not powder.

Make a habit of routinely preparing and eating vegetables from all groups to avoid becoming "Vegetable Resistant".™

NCD Pumpkin Shake™   NCD Steak & Eggs™

Choose God's version over man-made hybridized plants grown to produce fruit without seeds.™

Boycott fruits that have the words "Super Sweet" on them. They are just creating more diabetics by selectively hybridizing the plants to be high in sugar.™

Buy berries and other fruits during that 1-2 week window so you don't have to buy frozen or dried versions off-season.™

Consider drinking 1-2oz a day of Noni, Goji, Acai, or Mangosteen organic puree. See www.bioinnovations.net for their unique health benefits and deeply concentrated color.™

Always keep some Sunview organic raisins on hand for when you need a few extra carbs to go along with a meal.™

Since alcohol dehydrates your skin on the outside, imagine what it does on the inside. Moderation is Too Much.™

NCD Cantaloupe, Honeydew, and Watermelon juiced with rind.™

As you eat the foods you desire, and don't eat the foods you don't desire, over time you'll lose your desire for that food, and all foods, and simply eat to make your body perform, according to the needs of your Inner Divine Intelligence.

Make a plate of green beans, cooking them al dente, ¾ done, then snack on them like french fries.™

There's nothing nutritious about french fries, we just eat them because it's ingrained in our culture and our minds are on autopilot when we put them in our mouths.™

NCD Snap Peas is the easiest way to get a raw green vegetable.™

NCD Buffalo Chicken™   NCD Tuna Pasta Salad™

The NCD Washing Procedure for nonorganic produce is to use hot water and towel dry, three times.™

NCD Cherry Tomatoes, 3x12oz packs, aliquoted into nine 4oz servings, is an easy and excellent way to get a raw red.™

NCD Vegetable Sticks, carrots, celery, cucumber, organic zucchini, fit perfectly in the 8oz SKS jar. They look professionally prepared, provide extended expiration, and you'll enjoy eating them.™

Above all, when selecting produce, make sure that the skins are tight, no wrinkles, and the leaves are FRESH. Otherwise, pass.™

Eating spoiled or blemished produced causes more harm than good.™

Start your day with a handful of leafy greens, followed by a shot glass of Noni, Goji, Acai, or Mangosteen, to make even a bad day good.™

Triple-wash all leafy greens if you see suds or dirt.™

Adjust the thermostat of your refrigerator so that the internal temperature reads 0°C 32°F for extended food-expiration.™

Organic Spring Mix is the easiest way to get a leafy green, just pick it up at Walmart and eat it from the container.™

Switch to glass and join the growing number of Plastiphobes.™

For Clean Blood and a Clean Body, eat beets.™

Use any of the free vegetables to carry you to your next meal or to bedtime as a way to cut calories but still eat something.™

So, start your day with one of the leafy greens, then have a 4oz primary color, or a 3oz grapefruit, a T vegetable with a sprinkle of parmesan cheese, eating every 2-3-4 hours, recalibrating your body with X-country-ski walking, eating what you desire, according to your DI, becoming freed from food addictions, and taking control of your body weight and size by taking control of the numbers.™

NCD CLO Shot™

Only fish oil supplies the necessary DHA and EPA fats.™

Our ancestors took cod liver oil as part of their selfcare routine, but the next generations abandoned this good habit, hence the belief that most of us are deficient.™

DHA and EPA found in fish oil has become the number-one selling supplement on the market because of their, anti-inflammatory, blood pressure lowering, and improved circulation effects.™

Soft thick hair, lubed joints, and more energy are other effects.™

The marketplace has seen liquid fish oil replaced with capsules. This has led to the selling of small ineffective volumes, at 10x higher prices. The second reason for the change to capsules is to allow doctors to prescribe them to their patients.™

The benefits of fish oil happen when you "Go BIG".™

Cardiologists that recommend taking 8-10-12 or 14 capsules a day are in fact telling you to "Go BIG", but just in the wrong way, a way that benefit$ them more than you.™

When you buy fish oil, never mind the fancy versions. You take fish oil for the DHA and EPA. That's all.™

The NCD CLO Shot costs less-than $1, taken 10x per quarter or 40x per year = 48oz per year and only $36, or $3 per month. This is an effective annual amount and very affordable.™

In addition to its function in making flexible cell membranes, and organs such as the eyes, adrenals, testes, and brain, Omega-3 Flaxseed is our back-up "fish oil".™

Flax and Fish fats cannot be made by the body, we have to consume them. We have to "Seek Them Out" and have an action plan for doing so, otherwise, deficiency and its corresponding signs can occur.™

Could it be that all of the inflammatory diseases, high blood pressure, and circulatory problems, are simply due to a decades-long lack of dietary fish oil and omega-3 fat?™

Government and Industry are touting the benefits of omega-3, and warning us about trans fat, even outlawing it in some areas, and fish oil is the number-one selling supplement. Margarine is essentially illegal in New York diners. What does all this tell you?

The American People need to examine their current consumption of dietary fats and line them up with the information in this book.

NCD Fish Oil Rule, store it cold, take it at Room Temp.™

Don't waste precious time following those who are not themselves an example.™

The NCD is based on eating carbs, protein, and fat with each meal. The mixed-diet approach, three days of Atkins, one day of cheat, is just more nonsense and wasted time.™

"Cheating" has never made anyone successful long term.™

Separate yourself from the hype and easily-fooled masses of people out there. Be a clear-thinking individual. Discern the value of something before buying into it.™

History is always a good place to check. Does what you are being told pass the Time Test?™

Olestra (artificial fat) Time Test – Fail
Aspartame (artificial sweetener) Time Test – Fail
MSG (artificial flavor) Time Test – Fail
Hydrogenated Oils (artificial butter) Time Test – Fail
GMOs (artificial plants) Time Test – Fail
HFCS (artificial sugar) Time Test – Fail
BHA and BHToluene (artificial preservatives) Time Test – Fail

It's the "Slow Drip" method of assassination.™ One mouthful at a time. And the "Cocktail", a little of this, a little of that.™

Body Fat and Sugar Coating are two different weight gains.™

If you are lean and are overeating, you don't gain fat in the beginning because your excess calories are sugarcoating your cells. Keep it up and one day you will find, "Everything you eat turns to Fat." Your body is now saturated with sugar, Glycated.™

Now that you're overweight, you begin cutting calories to lose fat and it doesn't come off. Your body is burning off the sugarcoating first. But if you stick to it, one day you'll find, "The fat just starts melting off."™

Weight gain and weight loss are not something to be considered casually.™

Fat loss is tricky. Your body will resist you and your cravings for food will overcome you if you are not following a nutrition-based mathematical plan.™

Don't be fooled by shortcuts marketed by people with credentials and fame.   Often it's just another diet book rehashed and repackaged, with limited original content, and very little "Bridging" you to the results you want.™

Your body sees only three foods, protein, carbohydrate, and fat, and they add up to the "whole", calories, energy.™

Always check the label, especially the nutrition guides at fastfood restaurants, TF should always be 0.™

"Carb-Load" is an acceptable way to fill your muscles with fuel for the following days when you will work out.™

Of all "fast" foods available, 2% milk is the most macro balanced, about a third a third a third, and ~500 calories per quart. The NCD Emergency Meal.™

Your ancestors drank raw milk. Time Test – Pass

Raw milk provides the best Probiotics, gut flora, good bacteria.™

If you have any gastrointestinal problem, raw milk will fix it, or at the very least, make it less of a problem. The "danger" of raw milk is that it could eliminate your need for pills and scopes.™

The protein in raw milk has not been heated or denatured and the milk fat has not been spun into microlipid particles, bullets.™

321

Milk that costs $15 a gallon is a different product than milk that costs $3-4 a gallon. Just as canned cranberries are not the same food as fresh cranberries. Same words, very different products.™

If you are lactose intolerant, you likely have the gene that codes for lactase, however, your intolerance to milk is to the bad bacteria. Drink sterile milk by sterilizing it yourself, the NCD Milk Sterilization Procedure™, or buy UHT milk in the grocery aisle.™

The NCD recommends that you wean yourself back on to milk.™ The NCD Lactose Intolerance Protocol™ can help you do this.

Not only is "Good Milk Good Food" but it's also an alkalizer when it's metabolized.   So it's over there with the fruits and vegetables.™

Coffee and soft drinks are acidic, both pre and post metabolism.™

Three quarts of milk are about as alkalizing as drinking one quart of ABC Water™, about 3:1.

The lactose-intolerance campaign has resulted in several different product substitutions for milk, similar to the various designer varieties of fish oil. Just stick to the original version and you can't go wrong.™

If you made lactase as a baby, then you can still make it today.™

In all areas of life, Knowledge + Action = Results.™

God kept having her bring the book to work because He wanted Me to read it. I hope you see that He has put this book in your hands in much the same way.

Congratulations Winner ☙ !!   You passed the ABC NCD course!

Other Publications

Nontoxic Teeth Whitening and Dental Hygiene System
"Spare me the chemicals, I've switched to FOOD GRADE to
whiten, gargle and brush."

JPM Oral Hygiene Protocol
stop using toxic drugstore mouthwash, discover how to reduce
your gum pocket depth from 3-4-3 to 1-2-1 mm when they probe

NCD Flaxseed Shake Recipe
the Number Crunch Diet method for getting omega 3s
and with three variations so you'll never get bored

12 Changes A Year – Volume 1
the recipe book to the Number Crunch Diet
When you take control of the numbers you take
control of your weight.

The 5 Points of Posture
the missing link to fat loss, overall wellness, and
to becoming Respected, Adored, and Wealthy

12 Changes A Year – Volume 2
the recipe book to the Number Crunch Diet
Begin today and forever be in control of the numbers you're eating.

Vision Is Possible
Improve your vision and get a facelift for free!
an original vision program targeting your Eye Lids

The Author

I got my first job as a dishwasher at a steakhouse at the age of 14, back before there were laws regarding this. At 15, I moved up to Certified Broilerman. Still to this day I can cook a steak to MR doneness without having to cut into it to see. At 16 I bought my first car, the showroom Pontiac Sunbird, and paid cash for it. At the same time, I decided I wanted to be a dancer for a living and pushed forward with tap, jazz, and ballet classes, eventually dancing professionally, teaching, and choreographing, all of which allowed me to pay for my own university education.

My Bachelor of Science degree, left-brain education, balanced out my dance and arts, right-brain development, which, looking back, has given me a certain "whole holistic" view of things.

Later, I went back to university and became a Clinical Laboratory Scientist. These are the people that perform, report, and understand all those lab tests that people get when they enter a hospital. It is interesting to note that 70% of a typical patient's chart consists of clinical laboratory tests, performed by Clinical Laboratory Scientists. Whom most people have never even heard of, and yet our names are on 70% of all medical records, as the Performer/Reporter of those tests. I personally believe that no one understands lab tests better than a good CLS, we have all the technical information in our department.

During this part of my CLS career I delved into books one-after-the-other to understand health, wellness, and ailments more completely. As you know, there is traditional medicine, and then there is alternative medicine or holistic medicine, now being renamed complimentary medicine.

Fast-forward 20 years, and I now find myself at a point where it's time to publish all the discoveries, self-help material, and Revelation Information, that I've accumulated. If this book has benefited you, support my mission, and purchase a copy of this book for a friend or a relative. God Bless.

PREVIEW

As you know, the recipes for the NCD are being published under the titles, *12 Changes a Year* – the companion guide to the Number Crunch Diet. It may take up to a year to get them written as it will comprise about three volumes. In the meantime, you can get your pH paper testing set up and determine your current alkaline stores. The recipes read like a book and include additional information that I've discovered about diet, lifestyle, health and selfcare. I look forward to seeing you over there!

Jumper Publications & Media
from Advice to Results

CHAPTER 60

Follow-up

Yes, this chapter seems out of place, but, in a way not. I've referred to God, Jesus, and Angels in this book, and you can believe in them or not, either way is fine, but after 50 years of being on this planet, I can't deny their presence throughout my life. Hence, this chapter is Divinely provided.

There's a missing component to supplementing with bicarbonate in lieu of sufficient dietary fruits and vegetables, and that is, the question in the back of everyone's mind, "What if I'm taking too much?"

This is no different than any other nutrient. Too little is bad. Too much is equally bad. The word RANGE, needs to be added to your vocabulary. Laboratorians call it the Reference Range. The reference range for blood glucose is 70-110 mg/dL. For those of you in Canada, you use a different method for testing and so your range is 6-8, "six-to-eight feelin' great". Above 110 you are high, and above 400 you are critically-high. Below 70 you are low, and below 30 you are critically-low. So, Normal Range, outside of normal range, High or Low, and way outside of normal range, Critically-High and Critically-Low. Range Range Range. No matter what you take, whether it be iron, magnesium, calcium, you want to be in range range range. Too little iron results in too few red blood cells, anemia, and you have fatigue. Some athletes take iron to create more red blood cells, thinking that the more red blood cells the more oxygen and CO_2 exchange you get, resulting in better performance. I would never try that. Personally, I think it just makes for thick blood, too much hematocrit, (red blood cells), and not enough liquid-portion plasma.

Your body stores all these minerals and nutrients to varying degrees. Your pantry has lots of calcium on the shelves, but you don't want to use it, water-soluble vitamins B & C, not that much.

So what happened to me is, I stocked up my pantry shelves with alkaline, bicarbonate, this was wise, but I overstocked to the point that I had cases of bicarbonate stacked on the floor to the ceiling. Too much. You want to fill your pantry shelves with bicarbonate, (stock your alkaline reserves), but you don't want to overstock to the point where your shelves are full and so you have to start storing the extra in the walkway of your pantry. You get the idea.

I went over range with the bicarb. But this is great news because I now know what the signs are, and this is the reason for this chapter.

What to look for if you go over range.

1. My urine pH wasn't dropping.
Recall that your body is an acid-producing machine. How much depends on each individual. While writing this book, I stopped working out, hence, my acid production declined. Recall that the exerciser needs more bicarbonate, and the weightlifter needs a lot more bicarbonate. Heavy workouts plunge my urine pH. Bodybuilders, recall that you can speed your recovery and get your body fresh again after a workout by using ABC Water, Chapter 26.

So I wasn't working out, less acid production. Then, I didn't have time to make meals, so I switched to drinking 2% milk, 3 quarts a day, 1500 calories, equal to about 1 quart of ABC Water (milk is an alkalizer). So, no meat. Then it's spring, and I'm eating fresh in-season strawberries, then watermelon, then blueberries, and now mangoes.

Aside: It was just mango season, the last week of May, 2 for $1. I bought 18 mangoes for $9 and every one was delicious. Next week those mangoes will cost $1.49 each and will begin to have brown veins in them and you have to throw half of them in the trash. So I hope you are paying attention to your fruit windows. You only get one week a year for seasonal produce, or a month at most, to eat nutrient-rich fruits, that your body needs. (3 mangoes = ~500cal)

So, my lifestyle changed, no acid from working out, no acid from meat, alkalizing milk, and alkalizing fruit. Plus, I stuck with my one-quart-a-day-of-ABC-Water-religiously rule.

Here is the clue. Your body is constantly producing acid, so your urine pH should be constantly dropping. Mine wasn't. My urine pH was stuck at 7.0, with some 7.2s, and a few 7.4s. What's the rule? NO MORE ABC WATER FOR THE REST OF THE DAY, if you see a 7.2, and NO MORE ABC WATER FOR 24 HOURS OR LONGER, if you see a 7.4.

I broke my rule because I think God wanted me to experience what an overdose feels like so I can share it with my readers.

So clue #1 of overstocking your bicarb, i.e., your pantry shelves are full and your body has resorted to stacking bicarb on the floor, and up the wall to the ceiling, is:

YOUR URINE PH DOESN'T DROP

You should see your urine pH dropping because your body is constantly producing acid, how much, that depends on your diet, lifestyle, and emotions. Then you use the ABC Water to bump your urine pH up from 5 to 6 to 7, or from 6 to 7. If you prefer the 6.5 target, you bump your urine pH up from 5 to 6 to 6.5.

So, my urine pH stopped dropping. Clue #1.

Clue #2. Frontal Headaches. But not stress headaches, more like, amusement-park ride headache-rush headaches. Imagine being on a merry-go-round going round and round and then getting off and lying down on your back. Head Rush. Light Headed. That.

I would lie down to go to bed and I would feel lightheaded, like I had just gotten off of a merry-go-round.

Now, keep in mind, I have consumed about five cups of baking soda gradually over the past nine months. That's more than one quart of baking soda. So none of you are anywhere close to having had this amount.

In fact, here's what I would say about the adult population in general.

25% of the population likely has ¾^{ths} of a tank of bicarb. They feel fine.

50% of the population is likely around the half-tank mark, 40-60% full. These people probably have some problems or suspect something.

25% of the population is likely walking around with ¼th of a tank or less, they have overt health issues that they deal with daily.

ALL of these three groups of people, in my opinion, would benefit from taking ½ a cup of sodium-potassium bicarbonate gradually over the next 30 days to bump up their stores.

This would put the 3/4ths-tank people up to almost F, full.
This would bump the middle group up from 50% to ¾^{ths} of a tank.
And it would bump the quarter-tank people up to 40-50% of a tank, making them feel better, IN MY OPINION.

Since I have coined the term ALKALINE DEFICIENCY™, based on my personal experience, education, and knowledge, I believe this to be true. People on medication, NO. We already discussed that in Chapter 30.

If it took me five cups in nine months to overstock my pantry, a half a cup over 30 days would likely benefit the vast majority of the adult population, in my opinion.

Just like how they are saying we now need 5000 IUs of vitamin D and that the reference range is too low, and that you should take 10,000 IUs a day for 30 days to get stocked up, if your shelves are empty, you need to take extra to get stocked up. Recall Chapter 10, Stocking-Up Mode to Maintenance Mode.

Quite honestly, if I had been working out and eating meat, I would bet that I would not have gone above the range. But this is a good example of how your lifestyle affects your need for nutrients. My diet and lifestyle had changed to an alkaline diet and no-acid lifestyle, so I didn't need any ABC Water. Key Point to Remember.

But again, your urine pH is your indicator. Similar to how you would measure your blood pressure at home with a blood-pressure monitor, you have to look at the numbers and decide what to do. If your BP is 200/100 you probably want to take a pill and see your doctor. If your BP is 120/80, perfect, you're in range. If your BP is 100/60, uh-oh, too low!

Bicarbonate is a water softener. We already talked about this, and how it can soften the walls of your blood vessels. I am going to refer to bicarbonate as "blood pressure lowering". What happens if your blood pressure is too low, say, 100/60? Well, you feel lightheaded. You feel off-balance. You may not be able to feel your legs from the knees down. THERE'S NOT ENOUGH PRESSURE.

I personally believe that it's better to have higher blood pressure than lower. Slightly higher blood pressure creates a nice glow in your face and skin, whereas low blood pressure makes you feel weak, look pale, and can cause pooling in your extremities.

Now, any cardiologist will tell you that a diastolic, bottom number, greater-than 90 for more than two weeks requires diuretics, and I agree. The relaxation phase of your heart is not relaxing. Stress. Or stimulants. Coffee anyone? Green tea maybe?

I just don't think your systolic should be less-than 120, or 110 at the lowest, or you risk blood pooling at the extremities. My diastolic is 70-80, so I don't concern myself with the systolic. My systolic is a strong 125-145, but my diastolic phase is a calm and relaxed 70-80. Isn't the definition of healthy muscle tissue the ability to tense strong and then relax fully? I personally believe that a strong healthy vasculature is the kind that can tense hard and then relax fully. The medical system, as discussed before, is founded on their beliefs and models. You would be wiser to follow the fitness models and athlete's beliefs on health, and anyone who looks half their age. I've known my doctor for 20 years and visit him once every five years. He looks older each time I see him. I look about the same. This last time I saw him it had been five years. He looked old. I was shocked. He was equally shocked when he looked at me, because I still looked about the same. But the dictionary definition for looking half your age is Dr. Lorraine Day, www.drday.com. And there are others out there.

Let me take a moment to give another plug, endorsement. This book, I hope, will be read by fitness enthusiasts and people wanting to gain muscle, bodybuilders at any level. The person that helped me the most is Vince Delmonte, www.vincedelmontefitness.com. I bought his program for $77, which included like 3000 pages! I never read the menus, but I did read the book, *No Nonsense Muscle Building*. The book has real content, useful content. And, what impresses me is, you have to have lived it. Vince was skinny, now he's muscular, he wrote all of his own publications, he has a degree, and he built his business himself. He's authentic. Not a figurehead, actor, or spokesperson for a corporation, who's trying to sell you more empty fluff, nor a copycat of an original.

The new range for BP is now 120/80 to 90/60. While 90/60 may be okay for some people, for me, I would be flat-lining on the floor. There are 60,000 miles of blood vessels in the human body. I have probably double the vasculature of the average person. That would mean I have 120,000 miles of blood vessels. So I need a systolic BP of 125-145. I have twice the travel distance and roads to push through as the average person. When you get your blood drawn, the phlebotomist typically chooses from 3-4 veins. When the phlebotomist puts the tourniquet on my arm she quickly has to take it off or loosen it as I have 7-8 veins jumping out at her. I'm a phlebotomist's dream. She licks her lips and says "mmm", which one of these 7-8 juicy veins do I want to draw blood from. I have good healthy blood vessels, so I am not a believer that my blood pressure of 125-145 over 70-80 is "high". Personally, I believe your pulse is more important. If the average heart organ beats 3 billion times and then wears out, then a person with a 70 pulse, (beats per minute), will live to be 81.5 years old, and a person with a 50 pulse will live to be 114. But you won't hear the medical profession say much about pulse though. So set your pulse to 50.

Okay. I'll tell you how. Can you feel where the waist elastic on your underwear is? Breathe from there. Relax your ribs.

JPM – *The Five Points of Posture*

My point is, we are all unique. You are unique. My body's normal ranges and responses may not be the same as your body's normal ranges and responses. Science and the medical system would like to put us into little-box categories so it's easier to process us. Don't let them. You are Unique.

Clue #3. When I stood up from lying down, I would lose my balance. This progressed until it got to the point where I would stand up and I couldn't feel my lower legs below the knees. Low Blood Pressure.

Clue #4. I always wear a pulse watch. I bought mine at Walmart for $35, the Mio two-finger model. I also have the Sportline one-finger model. Both work good, I like the two-finger model better though. So what do you think happens when your blood isn't pumping back to the heart? Your Heart Beats Faster. Clue #4, your pulse goes up.

My pulse it typically 50 beats per minute. I like that. It's calm, cool, and collected. I am centered with a pulse of 50 and no one can push my buttons. I am unmoved by people and circumstances.

So buy a pulse watch and get to know your normal. This is another excellent device for the Selfcare Individual. Your pulse is a key to your heart. If it goes up, something's up. Upset? Caffeine? MSG? Or in this case, my pulse went up because my blood's not circulating because my vessel walls are too soft. Range Range Range. Too tense is too hard, too relaxed is too soft.

So my 50 pulse crept up to 60, then into the 70s, then 80, and then into the 90s on some occasions. Not good.

In summary then, the signs of too much bicarbonate are:
1. your urine pH doesn't drop
2. you get a merry-go-round head rush when you lie down
3. you don't have immediate balance when you stand up
4. your pulse goes up

Everything happens for a reason, and "all things work together for good". Romans 8.28

I stand by my statement – This Book is the Original Source Book for Determining Acid Alkaline Status and Correcting It.

You now have everything you need. Alkaline Deficiency and Alkaline Surplus.

Another thing you could do to prevent going over range, is to take your foot off the bicarb gas pedal one day a week and let your urine pH hit 5. In other words, just make sure you see one 5 per week. Or as a double precaution, two 5s. This is quite different than the person who has 35 urinations a week and 20 of them are in the 5s. That person is alkaline deficient in my opinion, see Chapter 10.

The person who is staying between 6 and 7, and then once a week skips the ABC Water just to be sure that their pantry is not overstocked with cases of bicarbonate on the floor going up to the ceiling because the shelves are full, this person is playing it smart.

So, Once A Week, Be Sure You See a Five.

That would be a good opportunity to notice how you feel. If you're like me, you may find that the ABC Water makes you feel so zoom zoom that you get kind of addicted to it, and then you start to "avoid 5 like the plague". So, as hard as it may be, allow your urine to bottom out to 5 once a week. See one 5 a week. Or, if you want to be doubly safe, two 5s a week, two 5s back-to-back on your off day. But definitely not 5-10-20 fives a week. That's deficiency.

As I grow with urine pH, it's likely there will be a Chapter 61 in the future. Be sure that I have your email address so I can email you additional chapters if and when they unfold.

abcwaterandthenumbercrunchdiet@mail.com

My target audience is the "Insider", the people running mini business empires, have a lot of responsibilities, stress (acid). My second audience is the exerciser. You'll never recover from a workout with a urine pH of 5. The third group are the people with overt health problems. You'll never get well with a urine pH of 5. I know the value of the information in this book. To help you further, I can provide you with the pH-paper system that I use. Just contact me at the address above. Many of you have more money than time. Why not skip the 4-day cruise and order the book and pH paper for all of your key people.

This is simple "Vehicle Maintenance" to keep you running.

Chapter Endnote
It seems I have more to say on acidosis, urine pH, ailments, and how they tie together. Chapter 61 will address this new "talk" about cancer patients having anger, and it's the anger that causes cancer. Not quite. As you know, anger is an acid-producing emotion. So it's not Anger=>Cancer, it's Anger=>Acid=>Cancer. Chapter 62 will look at the "bicarbonate" result on your laboratory chemistry panel for subtle clues, ask for copies of your lab results so you're ready. TCY will fill in the blanks for the Number Crunch Diet. See you there!

Leave a Review

Without giving away the contents, "spoilers", recommend this publication and leave a review so that someone else might benefit from it too. Thank you.

www.amazon.com   Search: Number Crunch Diet

Subscribe to my YouTube Channel
www.youtube.com   Search: Number Crunch Diet

Be sure to send me an email so I can periodically keep in touch with updates and new Selfcare Strategies – and discount offers on new items (yes, more than books!) (a simple and effective weight-loss device) (weightlifting "device" that I use EVERY time I work out) and don't forget the recipes! – TCY.

abcwaterandthenumbercrunchdiet@mail.com
Privacy – your email address will not be used for anything other than by Jumper Publication and Media.

Saliva vs Urine pH

Top Ten Reasons Why Saliva pH Is Worthless When Compared To Urine pH For Acid-Base Analysis

#10 Small Volume – small tiny volume samples don't represent the whole

#9 Difficult to Obtain – the procedure is to bring up saliva and swallow, 2x, then use the third one for the test, too hard to obtain

#8 Poor Reproducibility – when you retest your saliva sample, you will likely get a slightly different color (reading)

#7 Poor Accuracy – if you collect a second sample, it will likely give you a different reading than the first

#6 Bacterial Contamination – bacteria from your mouth will interfere with the test

#5 Food Contamination – food from your mouth will interfere with the test

#4 Spoon Contamination – the surface of the spoon that you collect it on is going to affect your small sample

#3 Viscosity – saliva is too thick and results in faded or dual colors of the test pad (or paper)

#2 Difficulty Reading – the color doesn't "lock in" so you can take a reading, it tends to change shades through a range

#1 Your Salivary Glands have ZERO to do with Acid-Base regulation. Try Kidneys.

Your kidneys are running your body's alkaline status.

And your alkaline status is the secret they don't want you to know.

Pick the correct answers – There may be more than one

1. A urine pH of 5 is telling you
   a. about your blood pressure
   b. that you're tired
   c. about your alkaline reserves
   d. to see a doctor
   e. that you're healthy and fine

2. Urine pH testing is routinely performed by licensed
   a. social workers
   b. clinical laboratory scientists
   c. respiratory therapists
   d. fitness advisors
   e. nurses and doctors

3. The cost of one month of urine pH testing is _____ the cost of
   open heart surgery (CABG).
   a. 1/10
   b. 1/100
   c. 1/1000
   d. 1/10,000
   e. 1/100,000

4. The opposite of metabolic acid is dietary
   a. phosphates – found in meats and cola drinks
   b. bicarbonate – found in packaged foods
   c. caffeine – found in green tea
   d. bicarbonate – found in fruits and vegetables
   e. bicarbonate – found in oils and fats

5. Information can be of which types
   a. true
   b. incomplete

c. false
d. clouded
e. secret

6. "Natural Flavor" on a food label is
   a. natural flavor extracts from plants and fruit
   b. glutamates, MSG, altered salts
   c. chemicals that make you addicted to the product
   d. generally safe and good for me
   e. not something I need to worry about

7. During World War II, the people who failed to act early
   a. suffered
   b. died
   c. lost everything
   d. became victims
   e. made it through unscathed

8. Compensating means
   a. saving for retirement
   b. eating foods that lift your mood
   c. doing something to mask something
   d. brushing it out of your thoughts
   e. pleasing others and being a do-gooder
   f. all of the above

9. The reason(s) people are fat
   a. they're born that way
   b. they don't make their own meals
   c. hereditary – handed down from your parents
   d. my body just won't lose fat
   e. they don't see the numbers in what they're eating

10. The "Cheat Day" is
    a. a great way to get food cravings satisfied
    b. required to reset my fat-burning hormones
    c. a 2-8 step backwards day
    d. works well for most people long term
    e. is a popular "trick" that you should buy into

ANSWERS

1. A urine pH of 5 is telling you
    a. about your blood pressure – No, but there is a relationship
       (see Chapter 24)
    b. that you're tired – No, but there is a relationship (see Chapter
       20)
    c. about your alkaline reserves – YES! Get to know your
       alkaline status by reading this book.
    d. to see a doctor – No, but it can lead to that.
    e. that you're healthy and fine – One number tells you little, 35
       numbers a week tells you a lot. Get to know your urine pH.

2. Urine pH testing is routinely performed by licensed
    a. social workers – no
    b. clinical laboratory scientists – Yes, 99% of all urine testing is
       done by a CLS.
    c. respiratory therapists – no
    d. fitness advisors – no
    e. nurses and doctors – Doctors do perform urine tests in their
       offices, but they are not looking at urine pH with much depth.

3. The cost of one month of urine pH testing is _____ the cost of
   open heart surgery (CABG)(a bypass, "cabbage").
    a. 1/10 – no
    b. 1/100 – no
    c. 1/1000 – no
    d. 1/10,000 – Yes. You can test all of your urinations for about

$1 a month (see Chapter 11). A cabbage would run you at least $10,000.
   e. 1/100,000 – no. But I believe the potential to save yourself $100,000 in medical treatments is very possible.

4. The opposite of metabolic acid is dietary
   a. phosphates – no, phosphates contribute to acidity
   b. bicarbonate – no, bicarbonate yes, but not from packaged foods
   c. caffeine – no, caffeine is a drug, most drugs are acidic
   d. bicarbonate found in fruits and vegetables – Yes!
   e. bicarbonate found in oils and fats – no, oils and fats are not sources of bicarbonate

5. Information can be of which types
   a. true – Yes, this is a bit what your life is all about. Finding the truth about things.
   b. incomplete – aka, partial truths or half truths, aka, "spin". Do you find your head spinning when you go for fancy medical treatments?
   c. false – lies, yes lies. Don't call them untruths. Lies are Lies. When people lie it's your job to call them on it. Otherwise, "ya got no backbone".
   d. clouded – blurry, muddied, confusion. I could write "scientifically" but I would just make you confused and half lost. How does that help you.
   e. secret – Now we're talking. When they say "buy this stock" you've got to be a moron to buy it. The payoffs and the winners are kept secret, shared through word of mouth.

6. "Natural Flavor" on a food label is
   a. natural flavor extracts from plants and fruit – Well, they would like you to think that, but that's far from reality.
   b. glutamates, MSG, altered salts – Yes, often this is the case.
   c. chemicals that make you addicted to the product – Yes

Absolutely
    d. generally safe and good for me – don't buy that line
    e. not something I need to worry about – you make your own choices in life

7. During World War II, the people that failed to act early
Referring to this is grim and bleak. But there are people suffering and dying every day because they failed to act early. You could say that WWII is still happening all around us in the United States of America today. My book can help you not to fall victim to this death and suffering. So that you make it through your life, unscathed.

8. Compensating means
    a. saving for retirement – no, but I have seen people who are just a little too attached to their portfolios, compensating?
    b. eating foods that lift your mood – no, but food is commonly used to compensate
    c. doing something to mask something – Ah-Ha, Yes.
    d. brushing it out of your thoughts – no. It's okay and healthy to let go of thoughts, just be sure you're not avoiding your issues.
    e. people pleasing – reward seekers may be compensating
    f. all of the above – no, just C. Go back and read C again.

9. The reason(s) people are fat
    a. they're born that way – don't give me that
    b. they don't make their own meals – Bingo! This is key.
    c. heredity – your fat jeans are because of your fat genes – no I don't think so
    d. my body just won't lose fat – I hear you. There is not a lot of good help out there. Luckily, you've found the right place.
    e. they don't see the numbers in what they're eating – Yes. And person D above just needs to look at food mathematically (and read the book).

10. The "Cheat Day" is
   a. a great way to get food cravings satisfied – Wrong. I'm a testimony of getting rid of food cravings. See Chapter 38, 39, 40, 41.
   b. required to reset my fat-burning hormones – Wrong. If you get your macros right, your hormones will cooperate just fine.
   c. a 2-8 step backwards day – On page 84 of *The Four Hour Body* the person states that he gains 4.4 lbs on his cheat day. Then he loses it. Can you say "moody"?
   d. works well for most people long term – After reading dozens of diet books, I could not find one that worked long term, so I made my own. It's called the Number Crunch Diet.
   e. a popular "trick" that you should buy into – The Number Crunch Diet isn't about cheating. Although it's full of useful "tricks" that I came up with and use daily.

You'll be miles ahead of the average person after a while.